Workbook

Introduction to
Medical
Terminology

by

Linda Stanhope
Health Science Department Head
Amarillo, TX

Kimberly Turnbull
Health Science Technology Instructor
Abilene, TX

Publisher
The Goodheart-Willcox Company, Inc.
Tinley Park, IL
www.g-w.com

Contents

The Basics and the Body

Name _____ Date _____

Understanding Word Parts

Answer the following questions.

1. What standard word parts make up most medical terms?

   _____

2. From which two languages do most medical terms derive?

   _____

3. What is the most commonly used combining vowel?

   _____

4. In general, when is a combining vowel *not* used?

   _____

   _____

5. The terms *dissect* and *dissection* are used several times in chapter 1. What do these terms mean? You may need to use a general dictionary or a medical dictionary to find their meanings.

   _____

   _____

6. What do medical terms ending in the letter combination *ae* signify?

   _____

   _____

Choose the correct plural form of each of the following terms.

_____ 7. appendix
   A. appendixes
   B. appendices
   C. appendicae
   D. appendicies

_____ 8. index
   A. indexaces
   B. indexi
   C. indexes
   D. indices

_____ 9. atrium
   A. atria
   B. atriumes
   C. atrium
   D. atriumies

_____ 10. bronchus
   A. bronchae
   B. bronchuses
   C. bronchi
   D. bronchies

(Continued)

Match each of the following word parts with the correct meaning. You will not use all of the meanings.

_____ 11. a-, an-

_____ 12. -algia

_____ 13. hyper-

_____ 14. -itis

_____ 15. trans-

_____ 16. inter-

_____ 17. -pathy

_____ 18. peri-

_____ 19. -oma

_____ 20. -ial

A. inflammation
B. between
C. across
D. pain
E. around; surrounding
F. not; without
G. tumor; mass
H. surgical repair
I. above; above normal; excessive
J. disease
K. pertaining to

_____ 21. cyt/o

_____ 22. path/o

_____ 23. gastr/o

_____ 24. super/o

_____ 25. cephal/o

_____ 26. arthr/o

_____ 27. my/o

_____ 28. lip/o

_____ 29. medi/o

_____ 30. ventr/o

A. above
B. muscle
C. middle
D. disease
E. heart
F. fat
G. cell
H. head
I. stomach
J. joint
K. belly side of body

Case Study—Medical Records and Abbreviations

Read the case study on page 2 of your textbook, and then define each of the following abbreviations.

Example

CBC: complete blood count

1. UA: _____

2. EKG: _____

3. CXR: _____

4. Pt: _____

5. NPO: _____

6. preop: _____

7. postop: _____

8. VS: _____

9. c/o: _____

10. abd: _____

11. SOB: _____

12. OB/GYN: _____

13. STAT: _____

14. b.i.d.: _____

15. Explain why healthcare organizations might use military time for their records.

_____

_____

_____

_____

_____

_____

_____

Anatomy and Physiology: Descriptive Terms

1. Explain the difference between the terms *anatomy* and *physiology*.

_____

_____

_____

_____

_____

_____

Write the correct term in each of the following paragraph's answer blanks.

The body is considered to be in the anatomical position when a person is standing _____
(2)
with the head and feet facing _____ , the arms at the _____ , and the palms
(3)   (4)
of the hands facing _____ .
(5)

Label the three planes in the following image.

6. _____

7. _____

8. _____

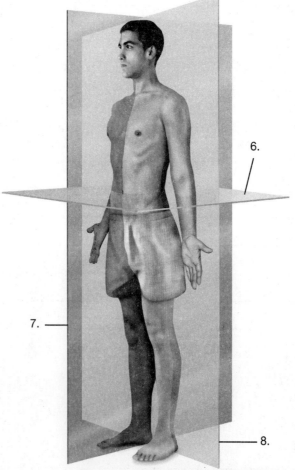

© Body Scientific International   *(Continued)*

Match each of the following body positions with the correct description. You will not use all of the descriptions.

_____ 9. erect

_____ 10. supine

_____ 11. prone

_____ 12. Fowler's position

_____ 13. Sims' position

_____ 14. lateral

_____ 15. knee-chest

A. a semi-sitting position, head of bed elevated
B. lying flat with the face down
C. left or right side; lying position
D. normal standing position
E. sitting up in a chair with head resting on a table in the front
F. lying flat with the face up
G. lying face down with knees bent while resting on the knees and chest
H. lying on side with hip and knee straight, and the other hip and knee bent or flexed

Match each of the following organs with the body cavity in which it is located. You will use some body cavities more than once.

_____ 16. heart

_____ 17. stomach

_____ 18. brain

_____ 19. urinary bladder

_____ 20. lungs

_____ 21. uterus

_____ 22. gallbladder

A. cranial cavity
B. thoracic cavity
C. abdominal cavity
D. pelvic cavity

Answer the following questions.

23. How would an anatomist (someone who is a specialist in the study of the structure of the body) define the term *hypochondriac*?

_____

_____

_____

24. Where is the epigastric region located?

_____

_____

_____

25. What does the term *hypogastric* mean?

_____

_____

_____

Body Organization

Answer the following questions.

1. Which term describes a state of physiological balance in the body?

   _____

2. Which term is used to describe the study of cells?

   _____

3. What is the "controlling" structure of the cell?

   _____

4. Which term describes a positive-charge ion?

   _____

5. Which term describes a negative-charge ion?

   _____

6. Define *pH*.

   _____

Match each of the following cell types with the correct description. You will not use all of the descriptions.

_____ 7. muscle cells	A. contains large, empty spaces
_____ 8. epithelial cells	B. long, with several fibrous extensions
_____ 9. fat cell	C. has a cell wall
_____ 10. nerve cells	D. long and slender
	E. flat and square

Complete the following statements by listing the three types of muscle cells, and then describing in which part of the body each type is found.

11. _____ muscle, attached to _____

12. _____ muscle, found in _____

13. _____ muscle, found in _____

(Continued)

Name _____ Date _____

Match each of the following organs with the body system in which it is located. You will use some body systems more than once. Some organs may be considered to be in more than one system.

_____ 14. lungs

_____ 15. bones

_____ 16. urinary bladder

_____ 17. trachea

_____ 18. spleen

_____ 19. heart

_____ 20. uterus

_____ 21. skin

_____ 22. joints

_____ 23. blood vessels

_____ 24. brain

_____ 25. testes

_____ 26. stomach

_____ 27. spinal cord

_____ 28. muscles

_____ 29. nasal cavity

_____ 30. pancreas

_____ 31. lymph nodes

_____ 32. kidney

_____ 33. tongue

_____ 34. prostate gland

_____ 35. ovaries

A. integumentary system

B. skeletal system

C. muscular system

D. nervous system

E. endocrine system

F. respiratory system

G. cardiovascular system

H. lymphatic system

I. digestive system

J. urinary system

K. male reproductive system

L. female reproductive system

Terms Related to Diseases, Conditions, and Assessment

Answer the following question.

1. Explain the difference between the terms *condition* and *disease*.

    _____

    _____

Complete each statement.

2. A nonrecurring, nonmalignant cancer is considered to be _____.

3. An abnormal growth, even if it is noncancerous, is called _____.

4. A temporary deficiency in blood flow to the brain is called a(n) _____ stroke.

5. A(n) _____ disease is inherited from one's biological parents.

6. A(n) _____ disease has a weakening or fatiguing effect.

7. A(n) _____ infection is acquired in a hospital setting and was not present upon admission.

8. A(n) _____ is the widespread outbreak of a disease that occurs within a country.

9. A condition that occurs as a result of a certain treatment, such as hair loss after chemotherapy for cancer treatment, is called _____.

10. The time period of recovery after an illness or injury is called _____.

11. A pathogen that normally does not cause disease in healthy people but may cause someone with a weakened immune system to get sick is called _____.

12. A disease that does not have any known cause is called a(n) _____ condition.

13. A(n) _____ condition occurs because of an external factor, such as trauma or an airborne virus.

14. A condition that is present at birth is called a(n) _____ disorder.

15. A(n) _____ is a set of signs or symptoms that occur together as part of a disease process.

(Continued)

Name _____ Date _____ _____

Match each of the following terms with the correct meaning. You will not use all of the meanings.

_____ 16. auscultation

_____ 17. diagnostic testing

_____ 18. inspection

_____ 19. manifestation

_____ 20. olfaction

_____ 21. palpation

_____ 22. percussion

_____ 23. prognosis

_____ 24. signs

_____ 25. symptoms

A. the use of smell to detect abnormalities

B. clinical presentation

C. the use of pressure on the skin above internal organs or structures

D. objective observations

E. the process of listening to body sounds using a stethoscope

F. a patient's record

G. prediction of the probable outcome of a condition

H. the use of lab tests, X-rays, and other diagnostic tools to identify a condition

I. a patient's awareness of abnormalities or discomfort

J. the process of observing one or more areas of the body

K. tapping on surface areas of the body to produce a vibrating sound

Chapter 1 Practice Test

Complete each statement.

1. Most medical terms are a combination of one or more basic _____.

2. A(n) _____ is a root word plus a combining vowel.

3. To learn medical terms, you may find it helpful to _____ a term down into its constituent parts.

4. The term _____ means "the study of disease."

5. In anatomy, the human body is divided into three imaginary flat sections called the
_____, _____, and _____
planes.

6. A(n) _____ is a space within the body that contains and protects internal organs and other body structures.

7. The _____ is the basic structural unit of the body.

8. A(n) _____ is a structure that is composed of several kinds of tissues working together to perform a specific function.

9. _____ the study of the causes of pathological conditions.

10. A(n) _____ is a shortened form of a medical term or phrase.

Using the word parts on pages 6–7 of your textbook, define the following medical terms.

11. gastritis: _____

_____

12. lipoma: _____

_____

13. biologist: _____

_____

14. thoracotomy: _____

_____

15. hepatomegaly: _____

_____

(Continued)

Name _____   Date _____

Using the word parts on pages 6–7 of your textbook, identify the medical term that corresponds to each of the following definitions.

16. a microorganism that produces disease: _____

17. a condition in which there is too much sugar in the blood: _____

18. a tumor of the connective tissue: _____

Identify the body system that corresponds to each of the following functions.

19. protects the body against microorganisms: _____

20. regulates body functions: _____

21. produces vitamin D: _____

22. transmits sensory messages: _____

23. filters airborne pollutants: _____

24. protects internal organs: _____

25. produces body heat: _____

26. carries chemical wastes to the kidneys: _____

27. removes solid wastes from the body: _____

28. facilitates survival of the species: _____

29. produces red blood cells: _____

30. filters blood to remove wastes: _____

List the most commonly used body position for each of the following procedures or goals.

31. chest X-ray: _____

32. preventing aspiration: _____

33. MRI scan: _____

Identify the abdominal quadrant in which each of the following organs is located.

RUQ   LUQ   RLQ   LLQ

34. left ovary: _____

35. stomach: _____

36. left ureter: _____

37. right fallopian tube: _____

38. gallbladder: _____

39. spleen: _____

40. right lobe of the liver: _____

(Continued)

Read the following medical record and then identify the meaning of the abbreviations that appear in bold. Refer to the table on page 23 and Appendix B on pages 427–431 of your textbook.

A 6 **y/o AAF** presents to **ER** with **c/o SOB** and wheezing on inspiration. Pt's caregiver states that she has had symptoms for several days and that symptoms have progressively worsened in the past 12 hours. **Pt** has a history of asthma. Caregiver reports that she has not been using her asthma medications for the past week because they "did not have the money to buy the medicine."

Assessment: Well developed, alert, and responsive. **wt**: 50 lbs; **ht**: 42 inches. **V/S WNL. NKDA**.

Orders: **STAT CXR, CBC. Consult** with Pediatric Pulmonologist and Social Services for assistance with asthma medication cost.

41. y/o: _____

42. AAF: _____

43. ER: _____

44. c/o: _____

45. SOB: _____

46. Pt: _____

47. wt: _____

48. ht: _____

49. V/S: _____

50. WNL: _____

51. NKDA: _____

52. STAT: _____

53. CXR: _____

54. CBC: _____

55. Consult: _____

Convert the following standard times to military time.

56. 1:15 p.m.: _____

57. 1:15 a.m.: _____

58. 10:45 p.m.: _____

Convert the following military times to standard time.

59. 2100: _____

60. 1330: _____

Chapter 2

The Skeletal System

Name _____ Date _____

Understanding Word Parts

Match each of the following word parts with the correct meaning. You will not use all of the meanings.

_____ 1. sub-

_____ 2. meta-

_____ 3. -algia

_____ 4. inter-

_____ 5. -itis

_____ 6. supra-

_____ 7. -al

_____ 8. intra-

_____ 9. -tomy

_____ 10. peri-

_____ 11. -penia

_____ 12. -malacia

A. above
B. within; in
C. inflammation
D. change; beyond
E. around
F. softening
G. process of cutting; incision
H. below
I. pain
J. between
K. abnormal condition
L. deficiency
M. pertaining to

_____ 13. oste/o

_____ 14. cervic/o

_____ 15. myel/o

_____ 16. arthr/o

_____ 17. ped/o

_____ 18. scoli/o

_____ 19. carp/o

_____ 20. synovi/o

_____ 21. tars/o

_____ 22. tendon/o

_____ 23. spondyl/o

_____ 24. orth/o

A. joint
B. wrist
C. crooked; bent
D. lubricating fluid of joints
E. bone
F. tendon
G. neck
H. foot; child
I. bone marrow
J. straight
K. vertebra; backbone
L. rib
M. ankle

(Continued)

Name _____ Date _____

Break down each medical term listed below by rewriting the term, and then placing a slash between each word part (prefix, root word, combining vowel, and suffix). Then define each term.

25. intercostal

    Breakdown: _____

    Define: _____

26. tendonitis

    Breakdown: _____

    Define: _____

27. kyphosis

    Breakdown: _____

    Define: _____

28. antipyretic

    Breakdown: _____

    Define: _____

29. arthralgia

    Breakdown: _____

    Define: _____

30. craniotomy

    Breakdown: _____

    Define: _____

31. arthroplasty

    Breakdown: _____

    Define: _____

32. rheumatoid

    Breakdown: _____

    Define: _____

33. subcostal

    Breakdown: _____

    Define: _____

34. lumbalgia

    Breakdown: _____

    Define: _____

35. narcosis

    Breakdown: _____

    Define: _____

Interpreting Medical Records

Use a regular dictionary or a medical dictionary to define the following terms.

1. aggravation: _____

2. alleviate: _____

3. therapeutic: _____

4. bulge: _____

5. In your own words, explain what *pain radiating* means. _____

6. What does the term *over-the-counter medication* mean? _____

Read the following medical record. Then define the abbreviations that are called out in the record.

Patient's Name: Jane Doe

ID Number: 12345

Date of Service: May 3, 2017

Subjective Data: 45 **y/o** female with **c/o** increasing difficulty using her **R** hand. **Pt** states she is "continually dropping things like her car keys and hairbrush." Pt states symptoms have worsened over the past six months. Pt states that she wakes up in the morning with severe numbness and tingling, and that it takes approximately two to three hours for symptoms to reduce in intensity. Pt's **OH** is a computer analyst for the past 20 years. Pt states that her **PCP** has ordered **OTC NSAID**s, occupational therapy evaluation with recommendations of home exercises, and night splinting. Pt states that symptoms have worsened despite conservative **Tx**. Pt referred to orthopedics for evaluation.

Objective Data: Pt is a well-developed female. **Ht**: 65 inches. **Wt**: 154.2 pounds. **HEENT** exam **WNL**. Evaluation of affected extremity reveals slight atrophy of R forearm in relationship to the L side. Wrist circumference: R: 18 **cm**, L: 19 cm. Pt is not able to distinguish between light and firm pinpoint pressures in the 2nd to 4th digits of the R hand.

Assessment: Moderate to severe **CTS**

Plan: Order **NCV** study. If this test indicates moderate to severe CTS, schedule Pt for endoscopic R carpal tunnel release. Instruct pt that if surgery is required, she will have to schedule to be off work for at least six weeks. If NCV study does not reveal CTS, contact Pt to return to clinic for further evaluation and Tx.

---

7. y/o: _____

8. c/o: _____

9. R: _____

10. Pt: _____

11. OH: _____

(Continued)

12. PCP: _____

13. OTC: _____

14. NSAID: _____

15. Tx: _____

16. ht: _____

17. wt: _____

18. HEENT: _____

19. WNL: _____

20. L: _____

21. cm: _____

22. CTS: _____

23. NCV: _____

Define the following terms.

24. orthopedics: _____

25. conservative treatment: _____

26. extremity: _____

27. digits: _____

28. endoscopy: _____

Answer the following questions.

29. Why do you think the patient described in this medical record developed CTS?

_____

_____

_____

_____

_____

30. What are some steps that patients can take to prevent or minimize this condition?

_____

_____

_____

_____

_____

Comprehending Anatomy and Physiology Terminology

Answer the following questions.

1. Explain the difference between the "axial" skeleton and the "appendicular" skeleton.

_____

_____

_____

_____

_____

_____

_____

_____

_____

_____

2. What are the five major functions of the skeletal system?

_____

_____

_____

_____

_____

_____

_____

_____

_____

_____

List one example of a bone in the human body that fits into each of the following categories of bone classification.

3. long: _____

4. short: _____

5. flat: _____

6. sesamoid: _____

7. irregular: _____

(Continued)

Name _____ Date _____

Label the different types of bones in the following image.

8. _____

9. _____

10. _____

11. _____

12. _____

13. _____

14. _____

15. _____

16. _____

17. _____

18. _____

19. _____

20. _____

21. _____

22. _____

23. _____

24. _____

25. _____

26. _____

27. _____

28. _____

29. _____

30. _____

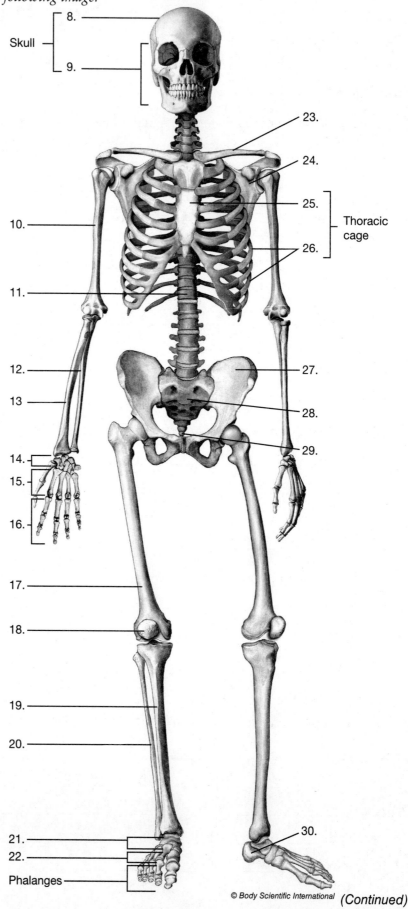

© Body Scientific International *(Continued)*

Answer the following questions.

31. What is the anatomical term for a bone's growth plate?

_____

32. Where is the periosteum located?

_____

33. What does the term *hematopoiesis* mean?

_____

34. What does the term *articulate* mean?

_____

Describe each type of joint and give an example of where each type is found in the body.

35. Diarthroses: _____

Example: _____

36. Amphiarthroses: _____

Example: _____

37. Synarthroses: _____

Example: _____

Match each of the following bone-related terms with the correct meaning. You will not use all of the meanings.

_____ 38. bone processes

_____ 39. tubercule

_____ 40. trochanter

_____ 41. tuberosity

_____ 42. condyle

_____ 43. bone depression

_____ 44. fossa

_____ 45. foramen

_____ 46. fissure

_____ 47. sulcus

_____ 48. sinus

_____ 49. suture

_____ 50. fontanel

A. opening or hollow region in the surface of a bone at a joint
B. shallow pit or cavity in or on a bone
C. passageway in a bone for blood vessels and nerves
D. one of two large processes found on the femur
E. a hollow cavity within a bone
F. areas on the bone that extend outward and serve as points of attachment for muscle or tendons
G. bones that form the floor of the cranium
H. deep, narrow, slit-like opening in a bone
I. point where cranial bones attach to each other
J. small, round process found on many bones
K. rounded knuckle process at a joint
L. soft spot on an infant's skull
M. large, round process found on many bones
N. a groove or furrow in a bone

Understanding Terms Related to Diseases and Conditions

Identify the term that corresponds to each disease or condition described below.

1. inflammation of the sac of fluid that is located near a joint:

    _____

2. a medical condition in which blood uric acid levels are elevated and can cause joint swelling and pain:

    _____

3. joint swelling at the base of the great toe due to inflammation:

    _____

4. luxation:

    _____

5. softening of the cartilage:

    _____

6. rheumatoid arthritis of the spine:

    _____

7. pain in the lower back:

    _____

8. inflammation of the covering that surrounds the bone:

    _____

9. inflammation of the bone and bone marrow:

    _____

10. rickets:

    _____

11. cancer of plasma cells:

    _____

12. partial dislocation of a bone:

    _____

13. clubfoot:

    _____

14. osteitis deformans:

    _____

(Continued)

Label each abnormal curvature of the spine shown in the following images.

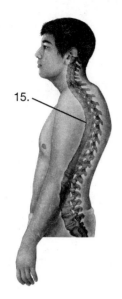

15.

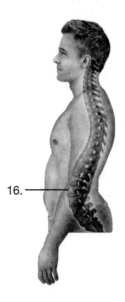

16.

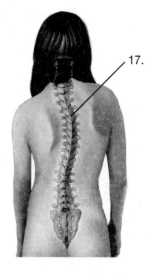

17.

© *Body Scientific International*

15. _____

16. _____

17. _____

Match each of the following terms related to fractures with the correct meaning. You will not use all of the meanings.

_____ 18. Colles fracture

_____ 19. comminuted fracture

_____ 20. greenstick fracture

_____ 21. oblique fracture

_____ 22. pathologic fracture

_____ 23. spiral fracture

_____ 24. stress fracture

_____ 25. compound fracture

A. a break across the bone at an angle

B. an open fracture

C. a fracture that may be a result of falling onto an outstretched hand

D. a break that is a result of a weakened bone

E. a common fracture seen in sports injuries

F. a fracture primarily seen in children

G. a fracture that splinters or crushes the bone

H. a closed fracture

I. a fracture that may occur because of an excessive impact

Analyzing Diagnostic- and Treatment-Related Terms

Identify the diagnostic test that would be considered in each of the following situations.

1. a test that may be used to collect cells that would be used in a stem cell transplant procedure:

_____

2. a test that is used to diagnose osteoporosis:

_____

3. a test that provides more detailed images than a regular X-ray but is not as costly as an MRI:

_____

Match each of the following surgical procedures or treatments with the correct meaning. You will not use all of the meanings.

_____ 4. arthrodesis

_____ 5. arthroplasty

_____ 6. physical therapy

_____ 7. diskectomy

_____ 8. bursectomy

_____ 9. amputation

_____ 10. traction

_____ 11. prosthesis

_____ 12. spondylosyndesis

_____ 13. ORIF

_____ 14. arthrocentesis

_____ 15. bone grafting

A. surgery to repair a fracture that requires the use of plates and screws

B. an artificial limb

C. the application of a pulling force to correct a dislocated shoulder

D. surgical immobilization of a joint

E. a procedure used to remove fluid from within a joint

F. the surgical fusion of vertebrae

G. the surgical removal of a vertebral disk

H. the straightening of a bone deformity

I. the surgical repair of a joint

J. the surgical removal of a limb

K. the process of rehabilitating a patient so that he or she is able to ambulate after hip replacement surgery

L. the process of transplanting and implanting bone tissue from the pelvic bones to repair a facial bone injury

M. the surgical removal of the sac of fluid that is found near the elbow joint

Using the word parts on pages 31–32 and Appendix A on pages 418–431 of your textbook, define the following medical terms.

16. subcostal: _____

17. bradykinesia: _____

18. arthrogram: _____

19. osteoarthritis: _____

20. pedal: _____

Preparing for Your Future in Healthcare

Define each of the following word parts that are related to healthcare professions.

1. chir/o: _____

2. neur/o: _____

3. muscul/o: _____

4. ultra-: _____

5. orth/o: _____

6. -ist: _____

7. radi/o: _____

Use the glossary in the back of the textbook or a dictionary to define the following terms.

8. manipulation:

_____

_____

_____

9. adjunctive:

_____

_____

_____

10. acupuncture:

_____

_____

_____

11. modification:

_____

_____

_____

12. intervention:

_____

_____

_____

(Continued)

13. customized:

_____

_____

_____

14. rehabilitation:

_____

_____

_____

15. amputation:

_____

_____

_____

Match the appropriate healthcare professional to each of the following tasks. You will use some of the healthcare professionals more than once.

A. chiropractor   C. orthopedic surgeon   E. radiologic technician

B. physical therapist   D. prosthetist

_____ 16. fabricates artificial limbs

_____ 17. educates people on exercises to improve their mobility

_____ 18. requires a DC degree

_____ 19. requires an MD or a DO degree

_____ 20. takes X-rays of bones

_____ 21. may use acupuncture as a treatment option

_____ 22. may work in a nursing home

_____ 23. is licensed to perform surgery

_____ 24. may practice with an associate's degree

_____ 25. must have a doctor's order before fitting a patient with a prosthesis

Chapter 2 Practice Test

Using the word parts on pages 31–32 of your textbook, identify the medical term that corresponds to each of the following definitions.

1. incision into the skull: _____

2. surgical repair of a joint: _____

3. pertaining to below the ribs: _____

4. inflammation of the bones in a joint: _____

5. resembling watery flow: _____

Break down each medical term listed below by rewriting the term, and then placing a slash between each word part (prefix, root word, combining vowel, and suffix). Then define each term.

6. subluxation

   Breakdown: _____

   Define: _____

7. osteopenia

   Breakdown: _____

   Define: _____

8. metatarsal

   Breakdown: _____

   Define: _____

9. intracranial

   Breakdown: _____

   Define: _____

10. arthodesis

    Breakdown: _____

    Define: _____

11. chondroma

    Breakdown: _____

    Define: _____

12. cranioplasty

    Breakdown: _____

    Define: _____

13. myeloma

    Breakdown: _____

    Define: _____

(Continued)

Name _____ Date _____

Label each of the following bones as either axial *or* appendicular *depending on which part of the skeletal system in which it is located.*

14. cervical vertebra: _____

15. clavicle: _____

16. frontal bone: _____

17. ribs: _____

18. fibula: _____

19. coccyx: _____

Answer the following questions.

20. Which two minerals are stored inside bones?

_____

21. Which structure attaches bones to muscles?

_____

22. Which term describes the shaft of a long bone?

_____

23. What substance is found at the edge of the growth plate that allows for new bone to form in children?

_____

24. Which term describes the hard, strong, and dense bone that forms the outermost layer of most bones?

_____

25. What is the smallest bone in the body? Where is it located?

_____

Identify the type of joint shown in each of the following images.

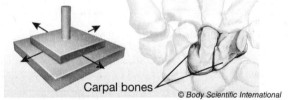

Carpal bones
© Body Scientific International

26. _____

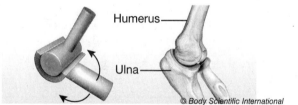

Humerus
Ulna
© Body Scientific International

29. _____

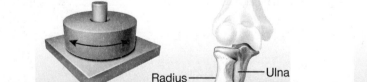

Radius ——— Ulna
© Body Scientific International

27. _____

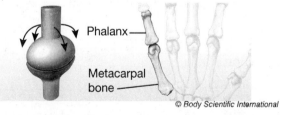

Phalanx
Metacarpal bone
© Body Scientific International

30. _____

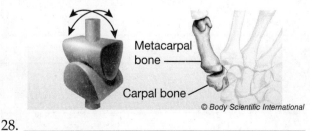

Metacarpal bone
Carpal bone
© Body Scientific International

28. _____

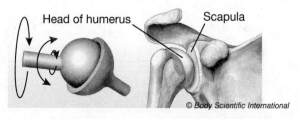

Head of humerus   Scapula
© Body Scientific International

31. _____

(Continued)

Name _____ Date _____

Identify the term that corresponds to each disease or condition described below.

32. inflammation of the sac that contains synovial fluid and is found between bones and muscles:

_____

33. inflammation of a joint that is caused by elevated levels of uric acid:

_____

34. a malignant tumor of the connective tissue that affects the bone:

_____

35. abnormal lateral (side-to-side) curvature of the spine:

_____

36. the partial dislocation of a joint:

_____

37. an abnormal depression of the sternum into the chest cavity:

_____

Identify the type of fracture shown in each of the following images.

© Body Scientific International

38. _____

© Body Scientific International

39. _____

© Body Scientific International

40. _____

© Body Scientific International

41. _____

© Body Scientific International

42. _____

© Body Scientific International

43. _____

© Body Scientific International

44. _____

© Body Scientific International

45. _____

Identify the term that corresponds to each treatment described below.

46. external manipulation to restore a fractured bone to the correct position: _____

47. the incision of a tendon: _____

48. the surgical repair of a bone: _____

(Continued)

49. the surgical removal of a vertebral disk: _____

50. the surgical repair of a joint: _____

51. the surgical removal of a limb: _____

52. an artificial limb: _____

53. the surgical repair of a fracture using hardware, such as pins and plates: _____

Identify the meaning of the bold abbreviation in each question below.

54. If a drug is ordered **PRN**, when would a patient take it?

_____

_____

55. If an arthroplasty were recommended because of **DJD**, what reason would you give the patient for the surgery?

_____

_____

56. If a drug is ordered **PO**, how should the patient take it?

_____

_____

57. If the doctor ordered a **BP**, what test would be performed?

_____

_____

58. If the medical chart states that the Pt c/o **LBP**, what problem does the patient have?

_____

_____

59. If a patient has a compound fracture, and the doctor is scheduling the patient for an **ORIF**, what kind of surgery will the patient be having?

_____

_____

60. If a patient's chart states that he or she was treated by the **ATT PHYS** at a hospital, what is that healthcare worker's title?

_____

_____

The Muscular System

Name _____ Date _____

Understanding Word Parts

Match each of the following word parts with the correct meaning. You will not use all of the meanings.

_____ 1. -esthesia

_____ 2. -plegia

_____ 3. brady-

_____ 4. -graphy

_____ 5. para-

_____ 6. -tonia

_____ 7. dys-

_____ 8. -dynia

_____ 9. -lysis

_____ 10. circum-

A. record; image
B. breakdown; separation
C. near; beside; alongside; beyond; abnormal
D. sensation
E. pain
F. slow
G. around
H. paralysis
I. tone; tension
J. process of recording
K. painful; difficult

_____ 11. tax/o

_____ 12. my/o

_____ 13. plant/o

_____ 14. son/o

_____ 15. orth/o

_____ 16. vers/o

_____ 17. rhabd/o

_____ 18. lei/o

_____ 19. kinesi/o

_____ 20. articul/o

A. straight; normal
B. smooth
C. muscle
D. tendon
E. sole of the foot
F. coordination; order
G. joint
H. sound
I. movement
J. rod shaped
K. turn; turning

Use the following combining forms listed on page 60–62 of your textbook to build the medical term that corresponds to each of the following definitions.

21. Word part: my/o

    Definition: breakdown of muscle tissue

    Term: _____

(Continued)

22. Word part: son/o

Definition: process of recording sound

Term: _____

23. Word part: fasci/o

Definition: incision into the fibrous band around a muscle

Term: _____

24. Word part: my/o

Definition: protrusion of a muscle through a tear

Term: _____

Break down each medical term listed below by rewriting the term, and then placing a slash between each word part (prefix, root word, combining vowel, and suffix). Then define each term.

25. dystrophy

Breakdown: _____

Define: _____

26. fibromyalgia

Breakdown: _____

Define: _____

27. neuromuscular

Breakdown: _____

Define: _____

28. myasthenia

Breakdown: _____

Define: _____

29. bradykinesia

Breakdown: _____

Define: _____

30. hemiplegic

Breakdown: _____

Define: _____

Interpreting Medical Records

Review the case study on page 60 of your textbook. Then use a regular or medical dictionary to define the following terms.

1. assessment: _____

2. posterior: _____

3. subsided: _____

4. therapeutic: _____

Read the following medical record. Define the abbreviations and terms called out in the record. Then answer the questions that follow.

University Rehabilitation Center

Physical Therapy Note

Patient's Name: Timmy Jones

Patient ID Number: 23456

Date of Service: January 12, 2017

Subjective Data: Pt is a 7 **y/o** male with **hx** of **DMD. Dx** was confirmed at age 3 by muscle **Bx** and **NMI**. Recent testing reveals a slight increase in muscular **hypertrophy** of the calves as compared to testing performed approximately 2 years ago. Pt's mother states that pt has increasingly **c/o** difficulty with **amb** and that he "just doesn't like to go outside and play with the neighborhood kids anymore." Pt's mother states that she continues to put his leg splints on at **hs**, but she has noticed that he will take them off during the night. She states that he c/o discomfort when the splints are on. Splints were customized for the Pt approximately 2 years ago. Pt's **PCP** has ordered **PT** evaluation and recommendations for **Tx** modalities.

Objective Data: Pt ambulates to exam table using an adjustable forearm orthopedic crutch, both **L** and **R** sides. Both crutches are extended to the maximum length. Pt's gait is waddling, **dystaxic**, and displays significant toe walking. Pt was able to get onto the exam table using upper extremities and with assistance from therapist.

Physical Exam: Upper extremity **ROM WNL**. Decreased ROM of **bilateral** lower extremities was observed. Also noted a marked decrease in **DTR**, lower extremities bilaterally.

Plan: Develop strengthening exercise program for outpatient PT 3 times a week for 6 weeks. Include **hydrotherapy** and **passive ROM** in Tx plan. Also develop and instruct Pt and mother on home exercise program, including **assisted ROM** to prevent **contractures**. Refer Pt to orthotics for custom fitting of new leg braces and rolling pediatric walker. Refer Pt to home health agency for occupational therapy evaluation and make recommendation for additional adaptive devices.

---

5. y/o: _____

6. hx: _____

7. DMD: _____

(Continued)

8. Dx: _____

9. Bx: _____

10. NMI: _____

11. c/o: _____

12. amb: _____

13. hs: _____

14. PCP: _____

15. PT: _____

16. Tx: _____

17. L: _____

18. R: _____

19. ROM: _____

20. WNL: _____

21. DTR: _____

Define the following medical terms that appeared in the medical record. Use the word parts lists, the information presented in chapter 3, and the glossary in the back of your textbook.

22. hypertrophy: _____

23. dystaxic: _____

24. bilateral: _____

25. hydrotherapy: _____

26. passive ROM: _____

27. assisted ROM: _____

28. contractures: _____

Answer the following questions.

29. Why do you think this patient doesn't like to walk anymore?

_____

_____

30. Why do you think this patient's leg splints are uncomfortable?

_____

_____

Name _____ Date _____

Comprehending Anatomy and Physiology Terminology

Answer the following questions.

1. List the six major functions of the muscular system.

_____

_____

_____

2. Skeletal muscle is also called _____ muscle.

3. Skeletal muscle fibers are held together with a structure called the _____.

4. Smooth muscle is also called _____ muscle.

5. The involuntary movement of smooth muscles is called _____.

6. Cardiac muscle is found in the _____.

Label the different types of muscles in the following image.

7. _____

8. _____

9. _____

10. _____

11. _____

12. _____

13. _____

14. _____

15. _____

16. _____

17. _____

18. _____

19. _____

20. _____

21. _____

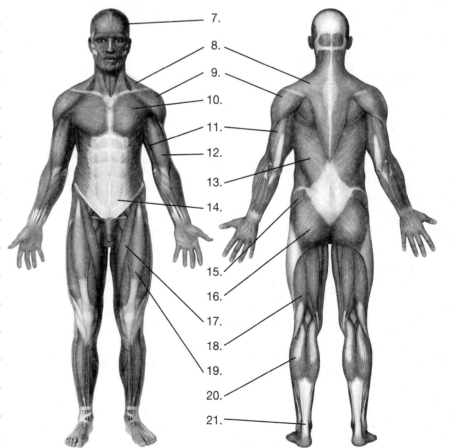

A. Anterior view   **B. Posterior view**

© Body Scientific International

(Continued)

Name _____ Date _____

Match each of the following descriptions with the correct term. You will not use all of the terms.

_____ 22. the site at which the muscle is attached to a bone that does not move when the muscle contracts

_____ 23. the band of fibrous tissue that connects a muscle to a bone

_____ 24. the ability of a skeletal muscle to contract

_____ 25. the ability of a skeletal muscle to receive and respond to a nerve impulse by contracting

_____ 26. the involuntary movement of smooth muscles

_____ 27. the ability of a muscle to contract without the involvement of nerves

_____ 28. the point of attachment of a muscle to a bone that moves during muscular contraction

_____ 29. the ability of a skeletal muscle to be stretched

_____ 30. the ability of skeletal muscle fibers to return to their original resting length

_____ 31. the band of fibrous tissue that connects a bone to another bone

A. automaticity

B. peristalsis

C. contractility

D. fascia

E. elasticity

F. tendon

G. origin

H. excitability

I. ligament

J. insertion

K. extensibility

Answer the following questions.

32. What term describes the movement of the feet when you are standing on "tiptoes" trying to reach something on a tall shelf?

_____

33. What term is used to describe your wrist movement when you reach out your hand to get some money from your parent?

_____

34. What is the position of your knees when you are sitting in a chair with your feet propped up on the coffee table in front of you?

_____

35. What term describes the movement of your left arm when you turn it with the right hand to look at the back side of your left upper arm?

_____

Understanding Terms Related to Diseases and Conditions

Answer the following questions.

1. What is a common complication that results from immobilization of or lack of use of a muscle?

   _____

2. Which gender is usually affected by DMD?

   _____

3. After a fracture is healed and the cast has been removed from an arm, the affected arm is generally smaller in size as compared to the unaffected arm. What term describes the condition of the affected arm?

   _____

4. In the case of a stroke, one side of the body is generally affected more than the other side. If there is total paralysis of one side of the body, what term describes this condition?

   _____

5. What term describes the condition that may affect the wrists of people who play video games for excessive amounts of time?

   _____

6. What two terms might you read in a medical chart describing a patient's c/o tenderness in the latissimus dorsi?

   _____

7. What term might an OB/GYN use to describe a benign tumor of the uterus?

   _____

8. Imagine that a day care worker has been sitting on the floor playing with the children for an hour. When she stands up, she experiences an uncomfortable sensation in her feet and lower legs. What term describes this sensation?

   _____

9. Parkinson's disease affects a patient's ability to ambulate. Terms used to describe the posture and gait of a patient with Parkinson's may include bradykinesia, a muscular stiffness called *rigidity*, and shuffling. One of the most prominent signs of Parkinson's is a quaking or shaking of the patient's limbs. What is the term used to describe this sign?

   _____

10. What does the term *hypertrophic cardiomyopathy* mean?

   _____

(Continued)

Name _____ Date _____

Break down each medical term listed below by rewriting the term, and then placing a slash between each word part (prefix, root word, combining vowel, and suffix). Then define each term.

11. plantar fasciitis

Breakdown: _____

Define: _____

12. rhabdomyoma

Breakdown: _____

Define: _____

13. hypothermia

Breakdown: _____

Define: _____

14. pathologist

Breakdown: _____

Define: _____

15. tendonitis

Breakdown: _____

Define: _____

Match each of the following descriptions with the correct term. You will not use all of the terms.

_____ 16. pain in a tendon

_____ 17. inflammation of a muscle

_____ 18. muscle pain

_____ 19. loss of muscle tone

_____ 20. muscle stiffness

_____ 21. softening of a muscle

_____ 22. stretching or tearing of a ligament

_____ 23. loss of muscle mass due to aging

_____ 24. stretching or tearing of a muscle

_____ 25. convulsive muscular contraction

A. sarcopenia
B. sprain
C. hypotonia
D. strain
E. myomalacia
F. tenalgia
G. myoparesis
H. myalgia
I. spasm
J. rigidity
K. myositis

Analyzing Diagnostic- and Treatment-Related Terms

Identify the diagnostic test that would be considered in each of the following situations.

1. a test to determine the involuntary response of a muscle:

   _____

2. a diagnostic testing method that will visualize soft tissue structures:

   _____

3. a test that measures the electrical activity of a muscle:

   _____

4. a test that uses sound waves to diagnose a leiomyoma:

   _____

Define each of the following abbreviations.

5. DMD: _____

6. RMS: _____

7. MD: _____

Suppose you are the sports trainer for your school. You have an athlete who has suffered a muscle injury. List the four steps involved in the most common first aid treatment for muscle injuries. Then, explain how you would teach the athlete what to do to continue the treatment when he or she gets home. Refer to the case studies on pages 60 and 86 of your textbook for additional information.

8. _____

9. _____

10. _____

11. _____

12. Home treatment:

   _____

   _____

   _____

   _____

   _____

   _____

(Continued)

Match each of the following descriptions of a therapeutic drug treatment with the correct term. You may match more than one term with each description.

_____ 13. treats pain

_____ 14. reduces inflammation

_____ 15. used to treat smooth muscle spasms

_____ 16. aspirin

_____ 17. includes OTC medications

_____ 18. may cause unconsciousness

_____ 19. may be used to treat a fever

A. analgesic

B. antispasmodic/anticholinergic

C. narcotic

D. NSAID

Use the table on page 81 and Appendix B on pages 427–431 of your textbook to answer the following questions.

20. The orthopedic surgeon has ordered an OTC analgesic to be taken PRN for pain postop arthroscopy. You are going to give the patient instructions for home management. When should you tell the patient to take a pain pill?

_____

21. A cake decorator has been having symptoms related to CTS. Her PCP has ordered her to wear R wrist splint hs. When will you tell the patient to wear the splint?

_____

22. You are the nurse on a hospital's orthopedic floor. Your pt is 4 days postop total knee replacement. The surgeon has ordered the intravenous line to be discontinued at 1300 (military time). The patient has been getting her pain meds intravenously. The doctor has ordered oral narcotics Q2-3H. At 1430, the patient requests "a pain pill." You quickly fill the order and give the patient the pill. When can you give the patient another pain pill?

_____

23. You are an ICU nurse taking care of a patient who has been in a car wreck. The patient was given CPR in the ambulance on the way to the hospital. Now, the patient is on a ventilator and not responding to verbal commands. The doctor has ordered you to perform DTR Q8H. Why would the doctor order this test for this patient?

_____

24. You are the pharmacist and a patient gives you a prescription for the NSAID naproxen 200 mg Q8H. The prescription explains that the patient has a drug allergy to PCN. The patient has been taking an OTC medication for stomach pains. To which medication is this patient allergic?

_____

25. You are a PFT working at a PT rehabilitation center. You have a new client who had back surgery three months ago and is trying to train for a marathon in six months. What is your job at the rehabilitation center?

_____

Preparing for Your Future in Healthcare

Define each of the following word parts related to healthcare professionals.

1. cardi/o: _____

2. myos/o: _____

3. radi/o: _____

4. -metry: _____

Use a dictionary or the glossary in the back of your textbook to define the following terms.

5. psychology:

_____

6. cardiopulmonary resuscitation:

_____

7. metabolism:

_____

8. musculoskeletal:

_____

9. rehabilitation:

_____

10. diathermy:

_____

Match the appropriate healthcare professional with each of the following descriptions or tasks. You may match more than one profession with each task. You will use each profession more than once.

A. certified fitness trainer   B. exercise physiologist   C. sports medicine physician

_____ 11. performs exercise stress tests

_____ 12. requires a MD or DO degree

_____ 13. does not require a college degree

_____ 14. may work with military pilots who are undergoing endurance training

_____ 15. may be the physician for a professional sports team

_____ 16. may work in clients' homes to develop personalized exercise programs

_____ 17. can prescribe medications

_____ 18. may teach yoga and Pilates at a fitness center

_____ 19. must have knowledge of the cardiovascular system to effectively develop a training program for clients

_____ 20. may perform surgery

Name _____ Date _____

Chapter 3 Practice Test

Use the word parts on pages 60–62 to build the medical term that corresponds to each of the following definitions.

1. incision into the fascia: _____

2. the process of bending: _____

3. record of sound: _____

4. muscle in the thigh that has four "heads" or attachments: _____

5. the study of the heart: _____

Break down each medical term listed below by rewriting the term, and then placing a slash between each word part (prefix, root word, combining vowel, and suffix if used). Then define each term.

6. kinesiology

Breakdown: _____

Define: _____

7. dorsiflexion

Breakdown: _____

Define: _____

8. dystaxia

Breakdown: _____

Define: _____

9. myodynia

Breakdown: _____

Define: _____

10. tenorrhexis

Breakdown: _____

Define: _____

Match each of the following muscles with the correct muscle type. You will use each muscle type more than once.

A. skeletal   B. smooth   C. cardiac

_____ 11. biceps femoris   _____ 16. vertebral column

_____ 12. urinary bladder   _____ 17. small intestines

_____ 13. larynx   _____ 18. right atrium of the heart

_____ 14. lungs   _____ 19. pectoralis major

_____ 15. left ventricle of the heart _____ 20. muscles around the lips

(Continued)

Identify each term being described below.

21. The term that describes the ability of the gastrocnemius to be stretched: _____

22. The term that describes the structure surrounding and binding muscle fibers into functional

    units: _____

23. The term used to describe the muscle that causes a body part's primary movement: _____

Identify the term that corresponds to each directional movement described below.

24. pointing the toes in a straight line away from the body, as when a ballerina stands on the tips of

    her toes: _____

25. moving one leg away from the other leg, as in getting up on a horse: _____

26. the rotational movement of the leg when the body is standing erect, the heels of the feet are as
    close together as possible, and the toes are pointing away from the midline of the body:

    _____

27. movement of the wrist when reaching over to pick up a pen from a desk: _____

Match each of the following muscle functions with the correct muscle. You will not use all of the muscles.

_____ 28. extends the forearm		A. gastrocnemius
_____ 29. flexes the thigh, extends the leg		B. biceps femoris
_____ 30. flexes the arm and forearm, supinates the hand		C. trapezius
_____ 31. raises the eyebrows; wrinkles the forehead		D. pectoralis major
_____ 32. flexes the foot and leg		E. gluteus maximus
_____ 33. dorsiflexes and inverts the foot		F. gluteus medius
_____ 34. extends the neck; elevates, adducts, and rotates the scapula		G. triceps brachii
_____ 35. extends and rotates the thigh		H. sartorius
_____ 36. abducts, flexes, extends, and rotates the arm		I. rectus femoris
_____ 37. flexes, adducts, and rotates the arm		J. latissimus dorsi
_____ 38. adducts and rotates the thigh		K. biceps brachii
_____ 39. extends, adducts, and rotates the arm		L. frontalis
_____ 40. flexes and rotates the thigh; flexes the leg		M. abdominal muscles
_____ 41. extends the thigh; flexes and rotates the leg		N. deltoid
		O. tibialis anterior

(Continued)

Identify the term that corresponds to each disease or condition described below.

42. total paralysis on one side of the body: _____

43. protrusion of a muscle through a tear: _____

44. loss of muscle mass due to aging: _____

45. inflammation of a muscle: _____

Identify the term that corresponds to each medical test or treatment described below.

46. measurement of the degree of motion of a joint in a variety of directions: _____

47. type of physical therapy in which a pool is used to decrease the amount of weight and impact on the joints: _____

48. the most common first aid treatment for muscular injuries: _____

Refer to the medical abbreviations on page 81 of your textbook to answer the following questions.

49. If a 79 y/o female is reported to have difficulty with amb, what problem does she have?

_____

50. If the doctor orders a patient to take an OTC analgesic postop, will this patient have to take a written prescription to the pharmacy?

_____

The Integumentary System

Name _____ Date _____

Understanding Word Parts

Match each of the following word parts with the correct meaning. You will not use all of the meanings.

_____ 1. epi-

_____ 2. -ectomy

_____ 3. sub-

_____ 4. -oma

_____ 5. auto-

_____ 6. -cyte

_____ 7. per-

_____ 8. -derma

_____ 9. -ose

_____ 10. -rrhea

A. cell
B. abnormal condition
C. tumor; mass
D. self
E. full of; pertaining to; sugar
F. flow; excessive discharge
G. on; over; upon
H. skin
I. surgical removal; excision
J. through
K. below

_____ 11. myc/o

_____ 12. blephar/o

_____ 13. xer/o

_____ 14. rhytid/o

_____ 15. hist/o

_____ 16. scler/o

_____ 17. ungu/o

_____ 18. cauter/o

_____ 19. steat/o

_____ 20. trich/o

A. hardening
B. fat
C. hair
D. nail
E. wrinkle
F. fungus
G. scale
H. tissue
I. dry
J. eyelid
K. heat; burn

(Continued)

Name _____ Date _____

Use the following combining forms and suffixes listed on pages 88–89 of your textbook to build the medical term that corresponds to each of the following definitions.

21. Word part: lip/o

    Definition: a mass of fat

    Term: _____

22. Word part: -osis

    Definition: abnormal condition of being bluish in color

    Term: _____

23. Word part: dermat/o

    Definition: inflammation of the skin

    Term: _____

24. Word part: -derma

    Definition: condition of hardening of the skin

    Term: _____

25. Word part: -esis

    Definition: condition of profuse sweating

    Term: _____

Break down each of the following medical terms by rewriting the term, and then placing a slash between each word part (prefix, root word, combining vowel, and suffix if used). Then define each term.

26. psoriasis

    Breakdown: _____

    Define: _____

27. immunology

    Breakdown: _____

    Define: _____

28. cryotherapy

    Breakdown: _____

    Define: _____

29. ecchymosis

    Breakdown: _____

    Define: _____

(Continued)

30. onychomyosis

    Breakdown: _____

    Define: _____

31. steatorrhea

    Breakdown: _____

    Define: _____

32. melanoma

    Breakdown: _____

    Define: _____

33. subcutaneous

    Breakdown: _____

    Define: _____

34. adipose

    Breakdown: _____

    Define: _____

35. xeroderma

    Breakdown: _____

    Define: _____

Name _____ Date _____

Interpreting Medical Records

Read the following medical records. Then define the abbreviations and answer the questions that follow each medical record.

A 27 **y/o** male presents to **ER** with second-degree burns to 9 percent of the lateral **RLE** as a result of a fire pit malfunction. **Tx** of the area includes irrigation with normal saline solution, applying silver sulfadiazine **oint**, and dressing the area with sterile gauze.

1. y/o:_____

2. ER: _____

3. RLE:_____

4. tx: _____

5. oint: _____

6. Explain where the burn was located.

   _____

   _____

A 60 y/o female presents to outpatient cosmetic surgery center to be evaluated for a possible face lift. **Pt** is a **NS**. Eval of **HEENT WNL**. Schedule this patient for rhytidectomy, bilateral blephroplasty, and dermabrasion. Explain to patient that these procedures are not covered by her insurance company because they are considered cosmetic.

7. Pt: _____

8. NS: _____

9. HEENT: _____

10. WNL: _____

11. Explain the three procedures listed in this medical record in terms that the patient would understand.

   _____

   _____

   _____

   _____

   _____

(Continued)

Pt is a 52 y/o male with an **OH** of outdoor construction work. Pt was seen by **PCP** due to **c/o** a lesion on the lobe of the **AS** that "just would not heal." **Bx** of site reveals Dx of basal cell carcinoma. Pt referred to dermatologist for possible Mohs surgery.

12. OH: _____

13. PCP:_____

14. c/o: _____

15. AS: _____

16. Bx: _____

17. Describe Mohs surgery.

_____

_____

_____

Pt has **hx** of excision of benign skin lesions, including a **cyst** in the **LLQ** of the **abd** area and a **nevus** on the R posterior lumbar area. 6-month **postop** evaluation shows the incision on the posterior lumbar area is a 2 cm x 0.2 cm well-healed cicatrix. The area on the anterior side reveals a 4 cm x 2.3 cm keloid. Pt states that this lesion is bothersome but denies pain. Recommend injecting the keloid with prednisone.

18. hx: _____

19. cyst: _____

20. LLQ: _____

21. abd: _____

22. nevus:_____

23. postop: _____

24. Explain the difference between a *cicatrix* and a *keloid*.

_____

_____

_____

_____

25. Where is this patient's keloid located?

_____

_____

Name _____ Date _____

Comprehending Anatomy and Physiology Terminology

Answer the following questions.

1. In its role as a physical barrier, what are three elements from which the skin protects the body?

_____

2. Explain how the skin helps regulate the body's internal temperature.

_____

3. What is the purpose of tactile receptors?

_____

4. Where would you find mucous membranes in the body?

_____

5. What does the term *stratified* mean?

_____

6. What does the term *squamous* mean?

_____

7. What three characteristics does connective tissue provide to the skin?

_____

Label the skin structures in the following image.

8. _____

9. _____

10. _____

11. _____

12. _____

13. _____

14. _____

15. _____

16. _____

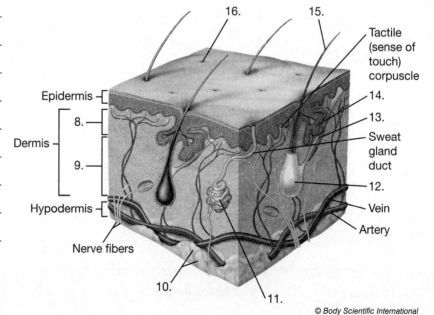

© Body Scientific International

(Continued)

Name _____ Date _____

Label the layers of skin in the following image.

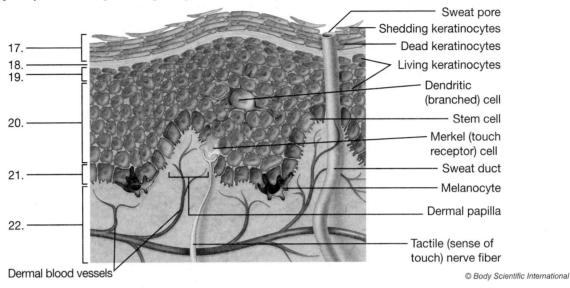

17. _____   20. _____

18. _____   21. _____

19. _____   22. _____

Answer the following questions.

23. Which layer of the skin contains the cells that store fat?

_____

24. What is the major difference between sebaceous glands and sweat glands?

_____

25. Where would you find the greatest amount of sweat glands in the body?

_____

26. Explain what causes the body odor associated with sweating.

_____

27. On average, who has more hair follicles, redheads or blonds?

_____

28. What causes someone's hair to "stand on end" when frightened?

_____

_____

29. What substance makes up the nails?

_____

30. Why should healthcare professionals look closely at the nails of the patients they are examining?

_____

_____

Understanding Terms Related to Diseases and Conditions

Answer the following questions.

1. What is the difference between impetigo and tinea?

   _____

   _____

   _____

   _____

2. A possible side effect of some medications, such as prednisone, is the occurrence of round, pin-point spots under the skin. What is the medical term for these spots?

   _____

3. Which condition causes the veins, usually in the lower extremities, to lose their elasticity and appear to be twisting?

   _____

4. What is the difference between a keloid and a wart?

   _____

   _____

   _____

   _____

5. How would you be able to visualize the difference between a case of psoriasis and a case of eczema?

   _____

   _____

6. Which chronic autoimmune condition may result in hardening of the connective tissue?

   _____

7. A symptom of an allergic reaction to a food or medication may be itching and the formation of hives. What medical term describes this condition?

   _____

8. Refer to the list of diseases and conditions on pages 94–98. Which two conditions are caused by poor blood circulation?

   _____

(Continued)

Name _____ Date _____

9. How do you determine if a burn is a first- or second-degree burn?

_____

_____

_____

_____

10. How do you determine if a burn is a second- or third-degree burn?

_____

_____

_____

_____

Match each description with the correct medical term. You will not use all of the terms.

_____ 11. small, raised skin lesion filled with clear fluid

_____ 12. crack or groove, as in a sore

_____ 13. smooth, slightly swollen area redder or paler than the surrounding skin

_____ 14. open sore or erosion of the skin

_____ 15. solid skin elevation with distinct borders

_____ 16. small, infected skin elevation that contains pus

_____ 17. closed, thick-walled sac containing fluid

_____ 18. small, flat, discolored lesion

_____ 19. skin elevation larger than one centimeter

_____ 20. highly pigmented lesion

A. macula
B. polyp
C. papule
D. nodule
E. wheal
F. vesicle
G. nevus
H. pustule
I. fissure
J. ulcer
K. cyst

Understanding Diagnostic- and Treatment-Related Terms

Answer the following questions.

1. Explain the difference between an allergy scratch test and an intradermal test.

   _____

   _____

   _____

   _____

2. A patient comes into the clinic with a possible basal cell carcinoma. What procedure may be performed to make sure this is the correct diagnosis?

   _____

3. The pathology report for the patient mentioned above came back as positive for basal cell carcinoma. The lesion is not very big or very deep. What might be the possible treatment to remove this cancer?

   _____

Imagine that you are a dermatology technician in a busy clinic. Answer the following questions using information you learned in chapter 4.

4. Your doctor is preparing to treat a young girl who has warts on her feet. Write an explanation you would give to the patient about what the doctor is going to do.

   _____

   _____

   _____

5. The next patient you are assisting the doctor with is having a cancerous growth removed from the right scapular area using the Mohs surgery technique. The patient has been prepared for the procedure, and the doctor makes the first incision before leaving the room. The patient seems worried. How will you explain what is happening to the patient?

   _____

   _____

   _____

6. Your next patient had sclerotherapy preformed a week ago. She is concerned that she cannot see a difference in her condition. How will you explain the healing process to your patient?

   _____

   _____

   _____

(Continued)

7. In the next room, a patient is waiting to have his second treatment of debridement after suffering from a third-degree burn on his left forearm. Last week, during the first treatment, the patient stated that his pain level was not as bad as he expected. However, the patient has noted that he is having more pain in the affected area, and he is concerned about the treatment today. He says he doesn't understand why he has to go through with this treatment today. How will you explain the purpose of this procedure?

   _____

   _____

8. You have relieved some of the burn patient's fears about the purpose of the debridement procedure, but he is still very apprehensive about the pain. What type of medication might the doctor give this patient prior to his procedure to help manage the pain?

   _____

9. During the debridement procedure, the doctor notes an area of possible infection. What type of medication might the doctor prescribe for this patient?

   _____

10. The next patient is a 4-year-old boy who has a severe rash due to poison ivy. His mother says that he can't sleep well because he keeps waking up feeling itchy. What type of medication might the doctor prescribe for this patient?

    _____

11. The next patient is a 26 y/o female who is undergoing removal of a tattoo on her posterior right shoulder area. This is her third session. What type of therapy would the doctor use for this procedure?

    _____

12. Next, the doctor will be performing an excision of a squamous cell carcinoma on a 72 y/o male. The doctor tells the patient that he will have to perform an autograft procedure. When the doctor leaves the room, the patient asks you what an "autograft" is. What will you tell this patient?

    _____

    _____

13. Your next scheduled patient is a 15 y/o male with tinea of the feet, bilaterally. What type of medication might the doctor prescribe for this patient?

    _____

14. The final patient of the day is a 55 y/o female with multiple skin tags in the neck area. What procedure will the doctor most likely perform to treat this skin condition?

    _____

15. Now you have some phone calls to return. Your last call is to a patient who has sought treatment for multiple skin cancers at your clinic. Yesterday, this patient visited an orthopedic specialist because he was complaining of back pain. The patient tells you that the orthopedic specialist gave him a transdermal pain medication called *Duragesic*. The patient is calling your office because he does not understand what the term *transdermal* means. He thought that you could explain how he is supposed to use this medication. What would you tell him?

    _____

    _____

    _____

Name _____ Date _____

Preparing for Your Future in Healthcare

Define the following word parts related to healthcare professions.

1. bi/o: _____

2. dermat/o: _____

3. path/o: _____

4. -dermis: _____

5. -ectomy: _____

Define the following medical terms related to healthcare professions.

6. dermatoplasty: _____

7. hypodermic: _____

8. onychectomy: _____

Answer the following questions using the information on page 105 in your textbook.

9. Of the three healthcare professionals mentioned, which one requires the most education?

_____

10. Which of these three professionals requires the least education?

_____

11. Which of these professionals can prescribe medications?

_____

12. Which of these professionals can perform surgery?

_____

For each of the professionals listed below, identify two or three possible facilities where the professional may work.

13. dermatologist:

_____

14. dermatology nurse practitioner:

_____

_____

15. dermatology technician:

_____

_____

Chapter 4 Practice Test

Using the word parts on pages 88–89 of your textbook, identify the medical term that corresponds to each of the following definitions.

1. removal of a nail:_____

2. a red (blood) cell:_____

3. the study of tissues: _____

4. treatment with cold:_____

5. inflammation of the eyelid:_____

6. inflammation of a gland: _____

7. the study of cells:_____

Use the following prefixes and suffixes listed on pages 88–89 to build the medical term that corresponds to each of the following definitions.

8. Word part: -osis

   Definition: the abnormal condition of dry, scaly skin

   Term:_____

9. Word part: par-

   Definition: an abnormal feeling or sensation

   Term:_____

10. Word part: -osis

    Definition: an abnormal condition of hardening

    Term: _____

11. Word part: -ic

    Definition: pertaining to death

    Term:_____

12. Word part: -osis

    Definition: an abnormal condition of blood in the tissues

    Term:_____

(Continued)

Name _____ Date _____

Break down each medical term listed below by rewriting the term, and then placing a slash between each word part (prefix, root word, combining vowel, and suffix if used). Then define each term.

13. hidradenitis

    Breakdown: _____

    Define: _____

14. erythematous

    Breakdown: _____

    Define: _____

15. pruritic

    Breakdown: _____

    Define: _____

16. trichomycosis

    Breakdown: _____

    Define: _____

Answer the following questions.

17. List the four major functions of the skin.

    _____

    _____

18. What is the term for the outermost layer of the skin?

    _____

19. What is the term for the cells that produce dark pigment in the skin?

    _____

20. Melanin is the pigment that gives skin its color. What is another important function of this pigment?

    _____

21. Which term describes the oil that is produced in the sebaceous glands and which helps to lubricate the hair and skin?

    _____

22. Which term that comes from the Greek word for "glue" is used to describe the connective tissue in the skin?

    _____

23. Which term describes the layer of skin where the fat cells are found?

    _____

(Continued)

24. Which term describes the half-moon-shaped structure that is found in the nail?

_____

Identify the term that corresponds to each disease or condition described below.

25. a burn that results in blisters: _____

26. bacterial infection common in children that includes vesicles, pustules, and crusted-over lesions:

_____

27. an abnormally raised and thickened scar: _____

28. hair loss: _____

29. a blister: _____

30. a freckle: _____

31. a small infected area of skin that contains pus: _____

Identify the term that corresponds to each treatment or procedure described below.

32. the destruction of tissue through heat, cold, or an electric current: _____

33. common treatment for the removal of basal cell tumors: _____

34. removal of damaged tissue to promote healing and prevent infections:_____

35. the procedure used to dissolve varicose veins: _____

The Blood and the Lymphatic and Immune Systems

Name _____ Date _____

Understanding Word Parts

Match each of the following word parts with the correct meaning. You will not use all of the meanings.

_____ 1. poly-

_____ 2. -lysis

_____ 3. -emic

_____ 4. -phage

_____ 5. meta-

_____ 6. trans-

_____ 7. -megaly

_____ 8. an-

_____ 9. -philia

_____ 10. -poiesis

A. not; without

B. enlargement

C. change; beyond

D. deficiency

E. love; attraction for

F. breakdown; separation; loosening

G. across

H. pertaining to blood condition

I. formation

J. many

K. eat; swallow

_____ 11. leuk/o

_____ 12. phleb/o

_____ 13. tox/o

_____ 14. hemat/o

_____ 15. lymphangi/o

_____ 16. iatr/o

_____ 17. erythr/o

_____ 18. tonsil/o

_____ 19. thromb/o

_____ 20. kary/o

A. red

B. blood

C. poison

D. vein

E. lymphatic vessel

F. vessel

G. nucleus

H. clot

I. tonsils

J. white

K. physician; treatment

(Continued)

Use the following combining forms and suffixes listed on pages 113–114 of your textbook to build the medical term that corresponds to each of the following definitions.

21. Word part: hemat/o

    Definition: formation of blood cells

    Term: _____

22. Word part: -logy

    Definition: study of shape or form

    Term: _____

23. Word part: hem/o

    Definition: bursting forth of blood

    Term: _____

24. Word part: hem/o

    Definition: stop the flow of blood

    Term: _____

25. Word part: -osis

    Definition: abnormal condition of a clot

    Term: _____

Break down each of the following medical terms by rewriting the term, and then placing a slash between each word part (prefix, root word, combining vowel, and suffix if used). Then define each term.

26. megakaryocyte

    Breakdown: _____

    Define: _____

27. phlebotomy

    Breakdown: _____

    Define: _____

28. thrombocytopenia

    Breakdown: _____

    Define: _____

29. metamorphosis

    Breakdown: _____

    Define: _____

(Continued)

30. serology

Breakdown: _____

Define: _____

31. neoplasm

Breakdown: _____

Define: _____

32. immunosuppression

Breakdown: _____

Define: _____

33. lymphoma

Breakdown: _____

Define: _____

34. hematocrit

Breakdown: _____

Define: _____

35. thrombolytic

Breakdown: _____

Define: _____

Interpreting Medical Records

Read the following medical record. Define the abbreviations and medical terms that are called out in the record. Then answer the question that follows.

PCP Services of Your Town USA

Patient Name: Sue Smith

Patient ID Number: 56789

Date of Exam: August 28, 2017

Subjective Data: **Pt** is a 58 **y/o** female with **c/o** increased fatigue x 3 weeks. Pt also reports that during her most recent **BSE**, she noted several swollen areas in her **R** and **L** armpit areas. Pt c/o slight tenderness. Denies redness or irritation on either side. Pt reports that her last mammography showed **bilateral** benign **fibrocystic breast changes**.

Medications: Multivitamins, fish oil capsules, calcium supplements, 81 **mg** aspirin every morning. Pt also takes **OTC NSAID PRN** for **LBP** and OTC omepraxole PRN for occasional **GERD** symptoms. Pt reports allergy to **PCN**.

SH: **NS**, has occasional glass of wine with dinner, denies recreational drug use.

OH: Recently retired school counselor

FH: Mother died at age 72 of breast cancer. Father died at age 76 of non-Hodgkins Lymphoma. Pt has one younger sister who is reportedly in good health. Pt has a twin sister who had a mastectomy approximately 3 years ago. Pt had older brother who died at age 54 of a **MI**.

Objective Data: Review of systems:

HEENT: Denies **HA**, dizziness. Reports **VA WNL**. No **lymphadenomegaly** noted in neck area.

Respiratory: Denies **SOB**. Lungs clear to auscultation.

CV: Denies chest pain, palpitations.

GI: Denies **dyspepsia**, **N/V**. Occasional c/o constipation, approximately twice a month.

GU: Denies dysuria or hematuria.

Neurological: Denies **syncope**, seizure, weakness, or **paresthesia**. **PERRLA**

Physical Assessment: **wt**: 165 pounds, **ht**: 64 inches

V/S: **T**: 98.6°, **R**: 14, **P**: 72, **BP**: 142/82

Axillary (armpit) area examined. R side: 2 swollen areas noted, consistent with lymph nodes. One measured 2.0 **cm** x 1.8 cm and medial to this one measured 1.2 cm x 1.2 cm. On the L axillary area, one swollen area noted. This area is more medial than the two on the R side. The lesion on the L side measures 2.5 cm x 2.3 cm. Pt verbalized slight discomfort upon palpation of these areas.

Plan:

Lab: **CBC**, **Hct**, **Hgb**, **WBC** with **diff**, **T**$_3$, **T**$_4$, **TSH**.

X-ray: **CXR**, mammogram, **CT** of bilateral axillary area to **R/O** lymphoma, breast cancer.

Define the following abbreviations that appeared in the medical record.

1. PCP: _____

2. Pt: _____

3. y/o: _____

4. c/o: _____

5. BSE: _____

6. R: _____

7. L: _____

8. mg: _____

(Continued)

9. OTC: _____

10. NSAID: _____

11. PRN: _____

12. LBP: _____

13. GERD: _____

14. PCN: _____

15. SH: _____

16. NS: _____

17. OH: _____

18. MI: _____

19. HEENT: _____

20. HA: _____

21. VA: _____

22. WNL: _____

23. SOB: _____

24. CV: _____

25. GI: _____

26. N/V: _____

27. GU: _____

28. PERRLA: _____

29. wt: _____

30. ht: _____

31. V/S: _____

32. T: _____

33. R: _____

34. P: _____

35. BP: _____

36. cm: _____

37. lab: _____

38. CBC: _____

39. Hct: _____

40. Hgb: _____

41. WBC: _____

42. diff: _____

43. T_3: _____

44. T_4: _____

45. TSH: _____

46. CXR: _____

47. CT: _____

48. R/O: _____

49. bilateral: _____

50. fibrocystic breast changes: _____

51. lymphadenomegaly: _____

52. dyspepsia: _____

53. syncope: _____

54. paresthesia: _____

55. Why do you think the healthcare provider suspected a possible diagnosis of cancer for this patient?

_____

_____

_____

Comprehending Anatomy and Physiology Terminology

Answer the following questions.

1. Name the two main fluids present in the body.

   _____

2. What two gases does the blood distribute to the cells and lungs?

   _____

3. What are the two major components of blood?

   _____

Using the word parts on pages 113–114 of your textbook, define the following medical terms.

4. erythrocyte: _____

5. thrombocyte: _____

6. hemoglobin: _____

7. polymorphonuclear: _____

8. hemolysis: _____

9. phagocytosis: _____

Match each of the following cell types with the correct meaning. You will not use all of the meanings.

_____ 10. albumin

_____ 11. basophil

_____ 12. erythrocyte

_____ 13. gamma globulin

_____ 14. lymphocyte

_____ 15. prothrombin

_____ 16. thrombocyte

A. contains histamine and heparin; also involved in inflammatory reactions

B. detects and destroys foreign cells

C. transports oxygen and carbon dioxide through the blood

D. aids in the process of blood clotting; also called a *blood platelet*

E. composed of proteins that act as antibodies

F. converted into thrombin in the event of an injury to a blood vessel

G. manufactures new blood cells

H. helps the body maintain proper fluid balance

(Continued)

Chapter 5   *The Blood and the Lymphatic and Immune Systems*   **67**

Name _____ Date _____

Label the structures of the lymphatic system in the following image.

17. _____

18. _____

19. _____

20. _____

21. _____

22. _____

23. _____

24. _____

25. _____

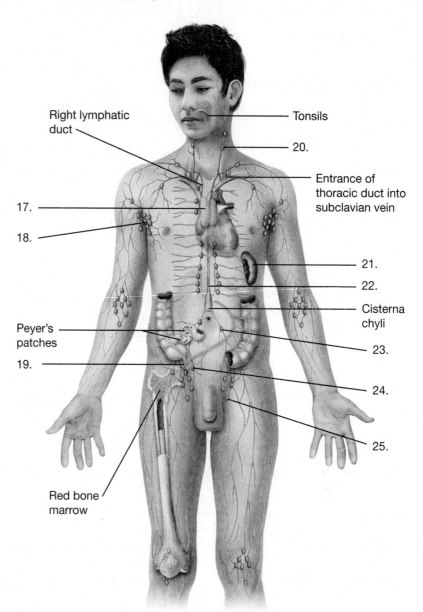

Right lymphatic duct

Tonsils

20.

Entrance of thoracic duct into subclavian vein

17.

18.

21.

22.

Cisterna chyli

23.

Peyer's patches

19.

24.

25.

Red bone marrow

© Body Scientific International

Match each of the following classes of B cells with the correct meaning. You will not use all of the meanings.

_____ 26. Immunoglobulin A

_____ 27. Immunoglobulin D

_____ 28. Immunoglobulin E

_____ 29. Immunoglobulin G

_____ 30. Immunoglobulin M

A. attaches to surface of B cells

B. acts as a powerful clotting agent

C. found in breast milk

D. targets sugars found in cancer cells

E. found in the respiratory tract

F. makes up 75% of all immunoglobulins

Name _____   Date _____

Understanding Terms Related to Diseases and Conditions

Match each of the following blood disorders with the correct meaning. You will not use all of the meanings.

_____ 1. aplastic anemia

_____ 2. hemolytic anemia

_____ 3. hemophilia

_____ 4. iron-deficient anemia

_____ 5. leukemia

_____ 6. multiple myeloma

_____ 7. pernicious anemia

_____ 8. polycythemia

_____ 9. sickle-cell anemia

_____ 10. thalassemia

A. deficiency of hemoglobin

B. deficiency of Vitamin B_{12}

C. failure of the bone marrow to produce enough blood cells

D. excessive production of RBCs

E. excessive destruction of erythrocytes

F. deficiency of thrombocytes

G. deficiency of iron

H. absence of a clotting protein in the blood

I. cancer of the bone marrow that results in uncontrolled growth of plasma cells

J. cancer of the bone marrow that results in increased amount of WBCs

Identify the term that corresponds to each of the classifications of diseases and conditions described below.

11. disease in which the body attacks itself, such as SLE and RA: _____

12. an infection that appears after someone has been in the hospital: _____

13. a condition with no known cause: _____

14. an allergy: _____

15. a condition that is present at birth: _____

16. a sudden outbreak of a contagious disease that affects a large group of people: _____

17. a new abnormal growth: _____

18. an infection caused by a microorganism that generally does not cause an infection unless someone's immune system has been weakened: _____

19. a condition or disease that has no cure and which will result in death: _____

20. the time period after someone has been sick but is improving: _____

Name _____ Date _____

Analyzing Diagnostic- and Treatment-Related Terms

Read the following scenarios and determine which test or medication would be used in each case.

1. Suppose you are the medical assistant at a primary care clinic. Your first patient of the day is Angela, a 16 y/o who is on her high school's swim team. She has been c/o being tired and unable to practice as long as she used to without resting. She has been experiencing heavy bleeding during her periods for the past 6 months. Her PCP is concerned that she may have anemia. The PCP has ordered a routine lab test to determine the number of RBCs, WBC diff, and platelets that Angela has in her system. You are going to fill out the lab request slip. Which test will you request for Angela?

_____

2. Imagine that you are a nurse in a busy ER. A gunshot victim is transported to your facility via ambulance. There is a large amount of blood on the gurney. The Hbg test in the ER shows that the pt's hemoglobin level is at 8 g/dL. You recall that normal hemoglobin values for men are 13.5 to 17.5 g/dL. You notify the attending ER doctor of the patient's hemoglobin levels. The doctor tells you to perform a test to check for blood-type compatibility on this patient. Which test will you identify on the lab request slip?

_____

3. The lab result on the test from the previous question shows that the patient has a blood type of AB positive. The ER doctor orders a procedure in which blood will be administered to the pt. You fill out the request slip for the blood bank. Which procedure will you order for this patient?

_____

4. Suppose you are the receptionist for an immunologist. Your physician hands you a lab request slip for a test to determine the levels of immunoglobulins present in a patient's blood. You are to verify that all the information is correct before you submit the request. What is the name of this test?

_____

5. Next, the doctor hands you a chart for a patient for whom he is recommending allergy shots to treat severe allergies. You are to make sure the insurance company will cover this procedure. What is the name of the procedure for which you will request preauthorization from the insurance company?

_____

6. The next patient who comes into the clinic has severe allergies and needs treatment because he is going out of town for a business meeting next week. The physician gives this patient an injection of Kenalog, a hormone-like drug that will decrease inflammation. You are completing the electronic chart to send to the patient's insurance company. What term will you use to describe the drug's classification?

_____

7. Imagine that you are the physician assistant (PA) working a night shift in a minor emergency clinic. A patient with a hx of sickle-cell anemia comes into your facility. The patient is c/o severe joint pain, SOB, and HA. You suspect that the patient is in a sickle-cell crisis. You order a test to determine the shape of the patient's RBCs. What is the name of this test?

_____

(Continued)

8. The next patient comes in c/o severe dysuria and hematuria. She states that she has had a fever between 100° and 102° for the past 2 days. She has taken OTC antipyretic medications such as acetaminophen, but the fever has not gone down. You suspect she has a UTI. You order a UA, which confirms your diagnosis. You order Bactrim, a drug that fights bacterial infections. What is this drug's classification?

   _____

9. Your next patient is a 17 y/o male who is the running back on his football team. He has a severe case of athlete's foot. He has been trying OTC products with no improvement in his symptoms of itching and burning. You give him a prescription for Clioquinol to treat his fungal infection. What is this drug's classification?

   _____

10. In the next exam room, you have a 28 y/o female who states that her 2 y/o daughter came home today with symptoms of the flu. Your patient is a busy executive, and she states, "I don't have time to get the flu." She explains that she had the flu vaccine about 3 months ago. You give her a prescription for Tamiflu to prevent and treat the viral infection of influenza. What is this drug's classification?

   _____

11. Suppose you are the oncology nurse at a cancer treatment center. The first patient of the day is a 58 y/o male. He recently had a procedure in which his dermatologist made an incision into a suspicious mole on his right posterior shoulder, removing a piece of the tissue and sending it to the pathology lab for examination. The patient wants to know the name of the procedure he received. What do you tell him?

   _____

12. The 58 y/o male patient was referred to oncology by his dermatologist because his test came back as malignant melanoma. You are to draw blood and send it to the lab for a series of tests. One of the tests will check for the ability of the patient's blood to clot. What is the name of this test?

   _____

13. The next patient you see in your office is a 55 y/o female who had a mastectomy due to breast cancer. She has undergone radiation therapy, and she is now ready to start the drug therapy of Methotrexate, which is used to prevent the growth of a neoplasm. What is this drug's classification?

   _____

14. The next patient is a 24 y/o male with a diagnosis of non-Hodgkin's lymphoma. You are to prepare him for a test in which a small amount of his bone marrow will be removed by a needle for evaluation. What is the name of this test?

   _____

15. In the next exam room, you have a 25 y/o female who has been receiving treatment for lymphoma for the past year. She is in the room with her 28 y/o sister, who has undergone testing and been approved as a perfect match for bone marrow donation. Your patient is excited and ready to have the procedure in which some of her sister's bone marrow will be injected into her body. Which term describes this procedure?

   _____

Preparing for Your Future in Healthcare

Using the word parts on pages 113–114 of your textbook, determine the area in which each of the following healthcare professionals specializes.

1. hematologist: _____

2. pathologist: _____

3. morphologist: _____

4. virologist: _____

5. cytologist: _____

6. serologist: _____

Define the following medical terms related to healthcare professions.

7. asthma:_____

8. eczema: _____

9. sinusitis: _____

10. prognosis: _____

11. biomonitoring: _____

Match the appropriate healthcare professional with each of the following descriptions or tasks. You will use each profession more than once.

    A. allergist/immunologist   B. epidemiologist   C. oncology nurse

_____ 12. may work at the CDC

_____ 13. can order and interpret medical tests

_____ 14. administers chemotherapy

_____ 15. requires a degree from a medical school

_____ 16. investigates how diseases are spread

_____ 17. develops treatment plans for patients

_____ 18. educates patients about home care

_____ 19. performs statistical analysis on information about diseases

_____ 20. works under the supervision of a physician

Chapter 5 Practice Test

Use a regular or medical dictionary, or the glossary at the back of your textbook, to define the following terms.

1. hemolysis: _____

2. splenomegaly: _____

3. antitoxin: _____

4. phlebitis: _____

5. thrombosis: _____

6. erythroblast: _____

7. fungal: _____

8. virologist: _____

9. metamorphosis: _____

10. phagocyte: _____

Use the combining forms and suffixes listed on pages 113–114 of your textbook to build the medical term that corresponds to each of the following definitions.

11. Word part: -ation

    Definition: process of clumping together

    Term: _____

12. Word part: -cyte

    Definition: cell with a large nucleus

    Term: _____

13. Word part: -plasm

    Definition: new formation/structure

    Term: _____

14. Word part: hem/a

    Definition: specialist in the study of blood

    Term: _____

15. Word part: -ical

    Definition: pertaining to the study of disease

    Term: _____

(Continued)

Chapter 5   *The Blood and the Lymphatic and Immune Systems*   **73**

Break down each medical term listed below by rewriting the term, and then placing a slash between each word part (prefix, root word, combining vowel, and suffix if used). Then define each term.

16. polymorphonuclear leukocyte

   Breakdown: _____

   Define: _____

17. fungology

   Breakdown: _____

   Define: _____

18. erythrocytopenia

   Breakdown: _____

   Define: _____

19. antineoplastic

   Breakdown: _____

   Define: _____

Answer the following questions.

20. List the three main types of cells in the blood.

   _____

   _____

   _____

21. Which term describes the type of immunity with which you were born?

   _____

22. Which term describes the condition caused by a lack of vitamin B_{12}?

   _____

23. Which term describes the condition in which a clotting protein is missing from the blood?

   _____

24. Why is mononucleosis called the *kissing disease*?

   _____

   _____

   _____

25. Which lab test examines the shape of red blood cells?

   _____

The Cardiovascular System

Name _____ Date _____

Understanding Word Parts

Match each of the following word parts with the correct meaning. You will not use all of the meanings.

_____	1. -emic	A. in; within
_____	2. brady-	B. above; above normal; excessive
_____	3. -tension	C. abnormal condition
_____	4. hyper-	D. pertaining to blood condition
_____	5. -stenosis	E. slow
_____	6. tachy-	F. fast
_____	7. endo-	G. pressure
_____	8. -sclerosis	H. to turn
_____	9. -ous	I. hardening; thickening
_____	10. -version	J. narrowing; tightening
		K. pertaining to

_____	11. dilat/o	A. lungs
_____	12. sept/o	B. narrowing
_____	13. coron/o	C. blue
_____	14. pulmon/o	D. clot
_____	15. systol/o	E. heart
_____	16. thromb/o	F. wall; partition
_____	17. angi/o	G. stretched; strained
_____	18. constrict/o	H. to enlarge or expand
_____	19. cyan/o	I. vessel
_____	20. tens/o	J. ventricle
		K. contraction

(Continued)

Use the following combining forms listed on pages 144–145 of your textbook to build the medical term that corresponds to each of the following definitions.

21. Word part: cardi/o

    Definition: inflammation within the heart

    Term: _____

22. Word part: angi/o

    Definition: record or image of a blood vessel

    Term: _____

23. Word part: cardi/o

    Definition: process of recording the electrical activity of the heart

    Term: _____

24. Word part: cardi/o

    Definition: tissue that surrounds the heart

    Term: _____

25. Word part: angi/o

    Definition: surgical repair of a blood vessel

    Term: _____

Break down each of the following medical terms by rewriting the term, and then placing a slash between each word part (prefix, root word, combining vowel, and suffix if used). Then define each term.

26. cardiomyopathy

    Breakdown: _____

    Define: _____

27. arteriosclerosis

    Breakdown: _____

    Define: _____

28. thrombophlebitis

    Breakdown: _____

    Define: _____

29. ventriculography

    Breakdown: _____

    Define: _____

(Continued)

30. cardioversion

   Breakdown: _____

   Define: _____

31. endoarterial

   Breakdown: _____

   Define: _____

32. anticoagulant

   Breakdown: _____

   Define: _____

33. echocardiogram

   Breakdown: _____

   Define: _____

34. cardiologist

   Breakdown: _____

   Define: _____

35. cardiopulmonary

   Breakdown: _____

   Define: _____

Interpreting Medical Records

Read the following medical record. Define the abbreviations that are called out in the record. Then answer the questions that follow.

County Cardiac Clinic

Patient Name: Harold Smith

Patient ID Number: 87654

Date of Exam: February 14, 2017

Subjective Data: **Pt** is a 67 **y/o** male **postop CABG** 6 weeks ago. Pt came into the clinic for evaluation for possible cardiac rehab orders. Pt denies any postop complications and states, "I haven't felt this good in years, except for the incision on my leg."

Medications:

Daily: Plavix 300 **mg PO**, Aspirin 325 mg PO, Fish Oil Capsules 1500 mg, Lipitor 50 mg, Lisinopril 25 mg

PRN: Nitrostat Sublingual 0.3 mg, take one when chest pain occurs. May repeat x3 doses. If chest pain continues, contact emergency medical services.

OH: Truck driver for interstate hauling company x45 years.

FH: Father died at age 65 of **CHF**. Mother died at age 82 of **CVA**.

Past Medical **Hx**: **HTN**; high cholesterol; obesity; smoker x25 years, quit approximately 2 years ago. Denies alcohol or recreational drug use. Admits to occasionally taking "energy" pills when he is on a long haul. Pt states that he normally eats fast food when he is out of town. He does not have a regular exercise program.

History of Present Illness: Pt states that approximately 2 months ago, he was out of town for his job and began having chest tightness, anxiety, sweating, and a feeling of "doom." He went to a minor emergency clinic in the town where he was staying, and was then referred to the **ER** at the local hospital. There he was evaluated for possible **MI**. Cardiac enzymes were elevated, and the **EKG** revealed ST-segment elevation. Pt was prepped for cardiac catheterization. Results of the catheterization showed 2 coronary artery lesions—one on the **LAD** artery and another on the **R** coronary artery. Angioplasty was attempted but was not successful due to the location of the plaque areas in the vessels. Patient requested to be allowed to travel to his hometown for further **tx**. Pt's wife was allowed to transport him back via private vehicle.

Pt was evaluated by his **PCP** and was immediately referred to **CV** department for evaluation of **Dx** of **CAD** and evaluation for possible CABG. Pt underwent this surgery and received 2 bypass grafts. Pt was discharged with skilled home nursing visits for continued monitoring x2 weeks. Pt's recovery period has been uneventful.

Pt states that he is trying to eat a more healthful diet and lower his cholesterol so that he can stop taking Lipitor. Pt states that he has lost almost 30 pounds since surgery, and that he is ready to get doctor's permission to start exercising.

Pt also reports that he has requested that his company transfer him to a local route so he will not be out of town for extended periods of time. He is planning on working for 2–3 more years, when he will be eligible for the maximum retirement benefits from this company. Pt states that he will have someone to help him with deliveries.

Physical Assessment: **wt**: 246 lbs, **ht**: 72 inches

V/S: **T**: 98.7°, **R**: 14, **P**: 90 **bpm**, **BP**: 150/92

(Continued)

Name _____ Date _____

> *Midsternal Incision*: 31.5 **cm** long. Well healed, some redness at the distal end. Pt states that pain in this area has subsided and only c/o occasional itching. Two incisions on **RLE** related to saphenous vein harvesting, medial proximal incision is 5.2 cm long. Second incision is 25 cm distal to previously mentioned incision. This distal incision is 4.5 cm long. Both incisions are slightly reddened; however, no discharge, warmth, or swelling has been noted. Pt states that these areas have been more worrisome than the incision on his chest.
>
> *Plan*:
>
> Refer patient to cardiac rehab program for cardiac monitoring during treadmill exercise. Frequency will be 3x week for 4 weeks and re-evaluation.
>
> Recommend that patient not lift anything over 10 pounds.
>
> Refer patient to dietitian for nutritional counseling and weight loss program.

1. Pt: _____

2. y/o: _____

3. postop: _____

4. CABG: _____

5. mg: _____

6. PO: _____

7. PRN: _____

8. OH: _____

9. FH: _____

10. CHF: _____

11. CVA: _____

12. Hx: _____

13. HTN: _____

14. ER: _____

15. MI: _____

16. EKG: _____

17. LAD: _____

18. R: _____

19. tx: _____

20. PCP: _____

21. CV: _____

22. Dx: _____

23. CAD: _____

24. wt: _____

25. ht: _____

26. V/S: _____

27. T: _____

28. R: _____

29. P: _____

30. bpm: _____

31. BP: _____

32. cm: _____

33. RLE: _____

34. What is the reason for the incision on this patient's leg?

_____

_____

35. What are some reasons that contribute to this patient's risk for developing heart problems?

_____

_____

Comprehending Anatomy and Physiology Terminology

Answer the following questions.

1. What is the primary purpose of the cardiovascular system?

    _____

    _____

2. Which terms describe the three layers of the heart?

    _____

3. Which term describes the upper chambers of the heart?

    _____

4. Which term describes the bottom chambers of the heart?

    _____

Match each of the following anatomical terms with the correct function or description. You will not use all of the functions/descriptions.

_____ 5. capillaries

_____ 6. veins

_____ 7. arteries

_____ 8. aorta

_____ 9. tricuspid valve

_____ 10. superior vena cava

_____ 11. pulmonary veins

_____ 12. aortic semilunar valve

_____ 13. inferior vena cava

_____ 14. pulmonary arteries

_____ 15. pulmonary semilunar valve

_____ 16. bicuspid mitral valve

A. located between the left ventricle and the aorta

B. carries oxygen-poor blood to the heart from the upper part of the body

C. general term that describes any blood vessel that carries oxygen-rich blood away from the heart

D. located between the left atrium and the left ventricle

E. the site where oxygen is delivered to the body's tissues and cells

F. located between the right ventricle and the pulmonary artery

G. structure that divides the heart into right and left sides

H. vein that carries oxygen-poor blood to the heart from the lower part of the body

I. general term that describes any blood vessel that carries oxygen-poor blood back toward the heart from the body

J. located between the right atrium and the right ventricle

K. blood vessel that carries blood away from the right ventricle into the pulmonary circulation system

L. the largest artery in the body, which carries oxygen-rich blood away from the heart into the systemic circulation system

M. blood vessel that carries blood from the lungs to the left atrium of the heart

(Continued)

Name _____   Date _____

Label the arterial pulse points in the following image.

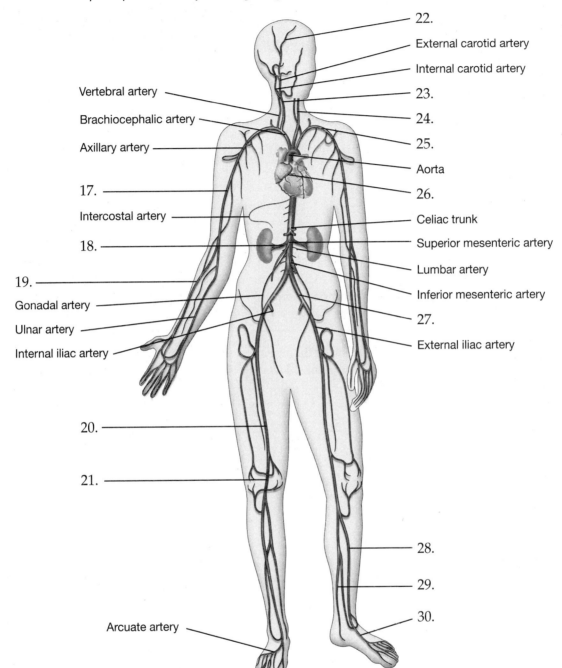

Vertebral artery

Brachiocephalic artery

Axillary artery

17.

Intercostal artery

18.

19.

Gonadal artery

Ulnar artery

Internal iliac artery

20.

21.

Arcuate artery

22.

External carotid artery

Internal carotid artery

23.

24.

25.

Aorta

26.

Celiac trunk

Superior mesenteric artery

Lumbar artery

Inferior mesenteric artery

27.

External iliac artery

28.

29.

30.

© *Body Scientific International*

17. _____   24. _____

18. _____   25. _____

19. _____   26. _____

20. _____   27. _____

21. _____   28. _____

22. _____   29. _____

23. _____   30. _____

Understanding Terms Related to Diseases and Conditions

Read the following scenarios and answer the question in each one.

For the following scenarios, suppose you are a nurse practitioner in a cardiology office.

1. The first patient you see has a pulse rate of 42 bpm. You know that a normal rate is between 60 and 100 bpm. How would you document this patient's heart rate?

   _____

2. The next patient has a resting heart rate of 125. How would you document this heart rate?

   _____

3. The next patient was booked as an urgent appointment. She has been complaining of pressure in her chest since 4:00 a.m. This patient was evaluated in the ER at 6:00 a.m. and was referred to your office. Which term would you use to document this patient's complaints of chest pain?

   _____

4. You schedule the previous patient for cardiac catheterization to determine if she has arteriosclerosis. She asks you to tell her what *arteriosclerosis* means. How do you describe this condition to her?

   _____

   _____

   _____

5. On your schedule, you see that your next patient has chronic CHF. What are some questions you will ask him to determine whether his condition is worsening?

   _____

   _____

6. When you examine the chronic CHF patient, you tell him that he has more cyanosis than normal. He asks you to explain what you mean. What do you tell him?

   _____

   _____

   _____

7. This patient's blood pressure is 90/45. You know that a normal blood pressure range is 90–140/60–90. Which condition would you document for this patient?

   _____

8. The medical assistant has already checked your next patient's blood pressure and recorded it as 170/96. Which condition would you document for this patient?

   _____

(Continued)

9. After your lunch break, the first patient you see has a new diagnosis of mitral valve prolapse. She asks you to explain this condition. How will you explain mitral valve prolapse?

_____

_____

_____

10. When you perform your examination on this patient with your stethoscope, you hear an abnormal sound. You know this sound occurs because the mitral valve is not closing completely. How would you document this in the medical record?

_____

11. Your last patient of the afternoon is a healthy, elderly patient who walks 3–5 miles every day. However, today he tells you that, in the past two weeks, he has not been able to walk more than half of a mile because he experiences pains in his calf. When he stops to rest, the pain goes away, but it comes back as soon as he starts walking again. What condition do you think this patient is experiencing?

_____

12. Which term will you use to describe your elderly patient's intermittent pain?

_____

For the following scenarios, suppose you are the charge nurse on the cardiac care wing of the hospital. You are reviewing the patient load so that you can assign patients to your incoming nurses for the evening shift.

13. In room 1421, you have Mr. Johnson, a 70 y/o male who was transferred to your floor from the Coronary Intensive Care Unit after having an angioplasty performed the day before. He has a diagnosis of CAD. You are going to instruct your nurse to teach this patient about CAD. How do you expect your nurse to describe this condition?

_____

_____

_____

14. In room 1412, you have Mrs. Rogers, who is 3 days postop for the repair of an abdominal aortic aneurysm. You are going to assign this patient to a nurse who just graduated from nursing school. How will you explain to this nurse the reason for the patient's surgery?

_____

_____

_____

15. In room 1423, you have Mrs. Smith, who was admitted from the ER earlier today with a blood clot in the vein of her lower left leg. The vein is inflamed, and the patient complains of pain in the extremity. What is this patient's likely diagnosis?

_____

(Continued)

16. Mr. Taylor is a 45 y/o male in room 1418 who is currently receiving intravenous antibiotic therapy to treat a bacterial infection that has caused inflammation of the inner layer of his heart. How would you document this patient's condition?

_____

17. You check the heart monitors of the patients on your floor and you notice that Mr. Jones in room 1415 has rapid, spontaneous contractions of the atria. You contact Mr. Jones' cardiologist with this information. How does the cardiologist describe Mr. Jones' condition?

_____

_____

_____

18. Later in the shift, you are visiting with the recent nursing school graduate, who is preparing to take the state board exam for his nursing license. He tells you that he has noticed his heart sometimes seems to have an irregular rhythm. You put an extra heart monitor on him and notice that he does have an extra, abnormal heartbeat that occasionally disrupts the regular ventricular rhythm of his heart. What condition does this nurse have?

_____

19. You have a nurse who tells you that she is going to be off work for the next few days to have her varicose veins removed. How can you verify that she has this condition?

_____

_____

_____

20. When you check on Mr. Johnson in room 1421, he tells you that the healthcare workers in the cardiac catheterization lab kept referring to his "MI." Since Mr. Johnson had been given sedation prior to the procedure, he could not remember what the healthcare workers told him about this condition. How do you explain to him what "MI" means?

_____

_____

_____

Name _____ Date _____

Analyzing Diagnostic- and Treatment-Related Terms

Match each of the following terms with the correct meaning. You will not use all of the meanings.

_____ 1. angiogram

_____ 2. auscultation

_____ 3. blood pressure

_____ 4. electrocardiogram

_____ 5. echocardiogram

_____ 6. nuclear ventriculography

_____ 7. exercise stress test

_____ 8. nuclear thallium stress test

_____ 9. stethoscope

_____ 10. Doppler ultrasound

_____ 11. cardiac catheterization

_____ 12. PET scan

_____ 13. sphygmomanometer

A. procedure in which a radioactive substance is injected into a vein near the end of a stress test to determine the sizes of the heart chambers, how well the heart is pumping blood, and if there is any tissue damage in the heart

B. the record of the electrical activity of the heart

C. test that uses a radioactive "tracer" to look for disease or poor blood flow in the heart

D. an instrument used to determine blood pressure

E. the process of listening to the internal body sounds

F. test that uses a "tracer" to measure the volume of blood that is pumped by the ventricles

G. a record or image of the blood flow in arteries or veins obtained by using a dye that can be visualized on a specialized camera

H. tool that is used to listen to internal body sounds

I. the procedure in which blood flow is measured using high-frequency sound waves

J. test in which a tiny plastic tube is inserted into a blood vessel, usually the femoral artery, to diagnose heart diseases or abnormalities

K. machine that continuously records the rhythm of the heart, usually for 24–48 hours

L. the measurement of a patient's cardiovascular health during exercise, usually on a treadmill

M. test that uses ultrasound technology to visualize the internal structures of the heart

N. term for the pressure exerted by the blood against the walls of a blood vessel

Identify the term that corresponds to each treatment method described below.

14. electrical device that is implanted in the chest to control abnormal cardiac rhythms:

_____

15. electrical device that is implanted in the chest to specifically control atrial or ventricular fibrillation:

_____

(Continued)

16. wire mesh tube that is inserted into an artery to prevent the artery from becoming blocked:

_____

17. procedure that sends controlled electrical shocks to the heart in a effort to restore normal cardiac rhythm:

_____

18. passageway that is established surgically, allowing blood to travel from the aorta to a branch of the coronary artery at a point beyond an obstruction:

_____

Match each of the following cardiac medications with the effect it has on the body. You will not use all of the definitions.

_____ 19. anticoagulant

_____ 20. thrombolytic

_____ 21. beta blocker

_____ 22. antianginal

_____ 23. diuretic

_____ 24. hypolipidemic

_____ 25. vasoconstrictor

_____ 26. antihypertensive

_____ 27. vasodilator

_____ 28. antiarrhythmic

_____ 29. ACE inhibitor

_____ 30. calcium channel blocker

A. helps reduce the amount of water in the body

B. prevents the formation of blood clots

C. dilates the arteries and reduces blood pressure

D. general term for any medication that is used to reduce blood pressure

E. prevents the body from making angiotensin II

F. stimulates widening of blood vessels

G. decreases inflammation

H. reduces lipid levels in the blood

I. prevents or reduces angina

J. used to treat several conditions, including angina, hypertension, irregular heart rhythms, migraines, panic attacks, and tremors

K. constricts or narrows blood vessels

L. prevents or reduces irregular rhythms of the heart

M. helps dissolve blood clots

Name _____ Date _____

Preparing for Your Future in Healthcare

Refer to the description of healthcare professionals on page 167 in your textbook. Then define the following terms. You may use the information in your textbook, a regular or medical dictionary, the glossary in the back of your textbook, and your own words to define the terms.

1. electrocardiogram: _____

   _____

2. sonography: _____

   _____

3. cardiac catheterization: _____

   _____

4. Holter monitor: _____

   _____

5. stress test: _____

   _____

6. cardioversion: _____

   _____

7. arrhythmia: _____

   _____

8. fibrillation: _____

   _____

9. defibrillation: _____

   _____

10. nuclear thallium stress test: _____

    _____

Match the appropriate healthcare professional with each of the following descriptions or tasks. You will use each profession more than once.

_____ 11. requires a medical degree

_____ 12. may supervise LPNs and CNAs

_____ 13. may work with physicians in a cardiac catheterization lab

_____ 14. can order heart testing for patients

_____ 15. monitors patient's heart rhythms while patient is in the hospital

A. cardiologist
B. cardiovascular technician
C. telemetry nurse

Chapter 6 Practice Test

Using the word parts on pages 144–145 of your textbook, define the following medical terms.

1. bradycardia: _____

_____

2. cardiomyopathy: _____

_____

3. thrombophlebitis: _____

_____

4. angioplasty: _____

_____

5. electrocardiologist: _____

_____

Use the following combining forms and suffixes listed on pages 144–145 of your textbook to build the medical term that corresponds to each of the following definitions.

6. Word part: angi/o

Definition: narrowing or tightening of a blood vessel

Term: _____

7. Word part: -ary

Definition: pertaining to the lungs

Term: _____

8. Word part: -ary

Definition: pertaining to the heart and lungs

Term: _____

9. Word part: -al

Definition: pertaining to the wall between the chambers of the heart

Term: _____

10. Word part: -ation

Definition: condition of excessive clotting

Term: _____

(Continued)

Name _____ Date _____

Break down each medical term listed below by rewriting the term, and then placing a slash between each word part (prefix, root word, combining vowel, and suffix if used). Then define each term.

11. septoplasty

   Breakdown: _____

   Define: _____

12. hypotrophy

   Breakdown: _____

   Define: _____

13. coagulopathy

   Breakdown: _____

   Define: _____

14. perivascular

   Breakdown: _____

   Define: _____

15. transvascular

   Breakdown: _____

   Define: _____

Answer the following questions.

16. Which term describes the sac that surrounds the heart?

   _____

17. Which term is used to identify the valve between the left atrium and the left ventricle?

   _____

18. Which term describes the sound heard through auscultation when the atrioventricular valves close?

   _____

19. Which term describes the structure in the nodal system where an electrical impulse terminates?

   _____

20. What is considered a normal systolic blood pressure range?

   _____

(Continued)

21. Where in the body would you find the popliteal artery?

_____

22. Which term describes the buildup of plaque in arteries that can lead to tissue damage in the heart?

_____

23. What is the term for a mass of plaque that travels through the bloodstream and can cause a blood vessel to become occluded, or obstructed?

_____

24. Which tool is used to measure blood pressure?

_____

25. Where on the body is a person's pulse detected?

_____

26. Which surgical procedure involves removing plaque from the lining of an artery?

_____

27. Which term describes the minimally invasive procedure in which a coronary artery is opened to allow better blood flow to the heart muscle?

_____

28. Which classification of drugs will help reduce the lipid (fat) levels in the blood?

_____

29. Which classification of drugs may be used to dissolve a thrombus?

_____

30. Which classification of drugs stimulates the widening of a blood vessel to maintain proper blood flow?

_____

Chapter 7

The Respiratory System

Name _____ Date _____

Understanding Word Parts

Match each of the following word parts with the correct meaning. You will not use all of the meanings.

_____ 1. dys-

_____ 2. eu-

_____ 3. -capnia

_____ 4. -thorax

_____ 5. -pnea

_____ 6. endo-

_____ 7. -tic

_____ 8. -phona

_____ 9. -stomy

_____ 10. -ectasis

A. flow; excessive discharge
B. voice
C. dilation; expansion
D. in; within
E. painful; difficult
F. pertaining to
G. breathing
H. carbon dioxide
I. good; normal
J. surgical opening
K. chest; pleural cavity

_____ 11. dilat/o

_____ 12. py/o

_____ 13. spir/o

_____ 14. ox/i

_____ 15. alveoli/o

_____ 16. bronch/o

_____ 17. sinus/o

_____ 18. pleur/o

_____ 19. rhin/o

_____ 20. carcin/o

A. nose
B. bronchial tube; bronchus
C. pleura; serous membrane that enfolds the lungs
D. air sac; alveolus
E. sinus; cavity
F. breathing
G. to enlarge; expand
H. oxygen
I. heart
J. cancer
K. pus

(Continued)

Use the following combining forms and suffixes listed on pages 175–176 of your textbook to build the medical term that corresponds to each of the following definitions.

21. Word part: bronch/o

    Definition: muscle contraction of a bronchial tube

    Term: _____

22. Word part: rhin/o

    Definition: condition of excessive discharge from the nose

    Term: _____

23. Word part: pneum/o

    Definition: condition of air in the chest, pleural space

    Term: _____

24. Word part: -ic

    Definition: pertaining to the diaphragm

    Term: _____

Break down each of the following medical terms by rewriting the term, and then placing a slash between each word part (prefix, root word, combining vowel, and suffix if used). Then define each term.

25. dysphonia

    Breakdown: _____

    Define: _____

26. tracheostomy

    Breakdown: _____

    Define: _____

27. bronchiectasis

    Breakdown: _____

    Define: _____

28. pyothorax

    Breakdown: _____

    Define: _____

29. spirometer

    Breakdown: _____

    Define: _____

30. thoracotomy

    Breakdown: _____

    Define: _____

Interpreting Medical Records

Read the following medical record and then identify the meanings of the abbreviations and medical terms that appear in bold. Refer to the table on page 197, Appendix B on pages 427–431, and the glossary in the back of your textbook. Then answer the questions that follow.

West Side ENT Clinic

Dictated by E. West, MD

Estella is a 3 **y/o** female with a history of chronic ear infections, allergic **rhinitis**, and **hypertrophy** of the tonsils and adenoids. She was referred to an **otorhinolaryngologist** for evaluation and **tx** recommendations. Pt's last tx for **tonsillitis** was 3 weeks ago. Strep test was negative. She was treated with Augmentin x 14 days.

Objective Data

General: Well-developed, well-nourished toddler. Responded adequately to age-appropriate commands.

GI: Pt's mother reports that Pt has a healthy appetite and normal bowel movements.

GU: Deferred

CV: heart sounds and rate **WNL** for age

Respiratory: Lungs clear to **auscultation**. No coughing or wheezing noted.

HEENT: **PERRLA**, denies **HA**, no gross abnormalities noted on external exam. No **lymphadenopathy** noted on **palpation** of posterior and anterior **cervical** lines. Pt is a mouth breather secondary to severe rhinitis. Tonsils are reddened, 3+ in size, and are crowding the **oropharyngeal** airway. Pt's mother confirms occasional **sleep apnea**, especially when Pt's allergy symptoms are severe. External ear canals are clean. Moderate bulging of the **tympanic membrane** is noted.

Recommendation: Schedule Pt for **tonsillectomy**, **adenoidectomy**, and **bilateral myringotomy** with placement of pressure-equalizing tubes.

Define the following abbreviations and terms that appeared in the medical record.

1. y/o: _____

2. rhinitis: _____

3. hypertrophy: _____

4. otorhinolaryngologist: _____

5. tx: _____

6. tonsillitis: _____

7. GI: _____

8. CV: _____

9. WNL: _____

10. auscultation: _____

(Continued)

11. HEENT: _____

12. PERRLA: _____

13. HA: _____

14. lymphadenopathy: _____

15. palpation: _____

16. cervical: _____

17. oropharyngeal: _____

18. sleep apnea: _____

19. tympanic membrane: _____

20. tonsillectomy: _____

21. adenoidectomy: _____

22. myringotomy: _____

Answer the following questions.

23. Where did the doctor check for swollen lymph nodes?

_____

_____

24. Why do you think this patient had occasional sleep apnea?

_____

_____

_____

_____

25. Refer to Figure 7.4 and the description of the pharynx and larynx on pages 180–181 of your text-book. Why do you think a nasal infection can lead to an ear infection?

_____

_____

_____

_____

Name _____   Date _____

Comprehending Anatomy and Physiology Terminology

Answer the following questions.

1. List the three main functions of the respiratory system.

    _____

2. Why do healthcare professionals usually measure a patient's respiratory rate after they measure the patient's pulse rate?

    _____

    _____

3. When a person suffers from an upper respiratory tract infection, which organs and structures may be affected?

    _____

4. Which structures in the vestibular region of the nasal cavities act as a first line of defense against infection?

    _____

Define the following anatomical terms, and then use these terms to label the diagram that follows.

5. nasopharynx: _____

6. oropharynx: _____

7. laryngopharynx: _____

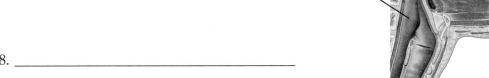

8. _____

9. _____

10. _____

Regions of the pharynx

© *Body Scientific International*

(Continued)

Answer the following questions.

11. What is the purpose of the epiglottis?

_____

_____

_____

12. What structures are considered to be part of the lower respiratory tract?

_____

_____

13. What does the term *ciliated* mean?

_____

_____

14. What does the term *bifurcate* mean?

_____

_____

15. In which respiratory structures does gas exchange occur?

_____

16. Which term describes the structure that separates the thoracic cavity from the abdominal cavity?

_____

17. Which term describes the watery membrane that surrounds the lungs?

_____

18. Which term describes the fluid found between the two membranes of the lungs that reduces friction during inhalation and exhalation to make breathing easier?

_____

19. Where is the control center that causes the diaphragm to contract, allowing air to flow into the lungs?

_____

20. The level of what substance in the blood determines the rate of respirations?

_____

Understanding Terms Related to Diseases and Conditions

Match each of the following medical terms with the correct meaning. You will not use all of the meanings.

_____ 1. orthopnea		A. a breathing pattern that is too slow and shallow
_____ 2. eupnea		B. a breathing pattern that is slower than normal
_____ 3. dyspnea		C. a temporary interruption of breathing
_____ 4. rales		D. a breathing pattern that is deeper than normal
_____ 5. hyperventilation		E. a breathing pattern that has periods of apnea followed by increased respirations
_____ 6. apnea		F. normal breathing
_____ 7. stridor		G. a condition in which breathing becomes easier if a patient is sitting up straight
_____ 8. hyperpnea		H. a breathing pattern that is labored, difficult, or painful
_____ 9. tachypnea		I. the term used to describe crackling sounds heard in the lungs
_____ 10. bradypnea		J. a breathing pattern that is faster and deeper than normal
_____ 11. rhonchi		K. a breathing pattern that is faster than normal
_____ 12. hypoventilation		L. the term used to describe coarse rattling or high-pitched snoring sounds heard in the lungs
		M. the term used to describe the harsh, high-pitched sound heard during inspiration

Read the following scenarios and answer the questions that follow.

> Imagine you are the nurse responsible for admitting patients into the ER. The first patient you see during your shift is a 20 y/o male who arrives via ambulance after being injured during a fight. He was stabbed in the left lateral side of the thoracic cavity. Air is now leaking into the pleural cavity.

13. What is the term for this condition?

_____

14. When the trauma surgeon evaluates this patient, she discovers that the knife severed several veins in the area. Now blood is leaking into the patient's pleural cavity. Which term describes this condition?

_____

(Continued)

The next patient is a 72 y/o male with a long history of smoking. He has been diagnosed with a chronic pulmonary disease in which the alveoli are larger than normal and have lost their elasticity.

15. What diagnosis will you record on this patient's admission form?

   _____

16. This patient's PCP recently told him that his lung function has worsened. His lungs' ability to perform their function of ventilation has been reduced, and he now has less than 50 percent normal inspiratory capacity based on his last pulmonary function test. Given this information, what additional diagnosis will you include on this patient's admission form?

   _____

The next patient is Amy, a 7 y/o female who comes into the ER with c/o increased dyspnea. Her mother reports that Amy was playing outside earlier today while her neighbor was mowing the lawn. When Amy came into the house, her eyes were reddened and she had severe rhinorrhea. Amy told her mother that she could not breathe through her nose. Her mother says that the mucous membranes in Amy's nose were swollen and red.

17. What diagnosis would you record in Amy's chart?

   _____

18. When you perform auscultation of Amy's lungs, you notice a definite wheezing sound during respiration. You know that this sound is made when there is a swelling or spasm of the bronchial tubes. What additional diagnosis do you now suspect for Amy?

   _____

Your next patient is Bobby, a 12 y/o male who c/o a sore throat. Upon examination of this patient, you notice that his tonsils are extremely inflamed.

19. What is the medical term for this condition?

   _____

20. The ER doctor performs a test that confirms the presence of the bacterium *Streptococcus*. What diagnosis do you think matches Bobby's condition?

   _____

Analyzing Diagnostic- and Treatment-Related Terms

Answer the question in each of the following scenarios.

1. Your grandma has been complaining that your grandpa snores so loudly it keeps her up at night. Your grandpa agrees to see the doctor because he has not been sleeping well either. The doctor orders a test to determine if your grandpa has sleep apnea. What is the name of this test?

   _____

2. If your grandpa is diagnosed with sleep apnea, he may receive treatment that includes wearing a mask attached to a machine that delivers mild air pressure to keep his airways open while he sleeps. What is the name for this treatment method?

   _____

3. Your aunt is a nurse's aide in a long-term skilled nursing facility. She tells you about a test that she had to have completed before she could work there. This test required her to have a small amount of a certain purified protein derivative injected under the skin of her forearm. She had to go back to the doctor's office 48–72 hours after the injection to see if there was any reaction to the derivative. What is the name of this test?

   _____

4. Your best friend's dad went to the doctor recently because he had a cough for about two weeks. The doctor suspects a diagnosis of pneumonia. What radiographic test might the doctor order to obtain images of the anterior, posterior, and lateral views of the lungs?

   _____

5. If the test mentioned in the previous question confirms that your friend's dad has pneumonia, the doctor may order another test. This test would determine which bacteria is growing in the lung secretions, as well as which antibiotic would most effectively treat the infection. What is the name of this test?

   _____

6. This test confirms that your friend's dad has bacterial pneumonia. What medication might the doctor prescribe to treat this infection?

   _____

7. You notice that you haven't seen your neighbor, Mr. Smith, out in his yard for several weeks. He used to stand on the front porch every night to smoke. When you next see Mrs. Smith, you ask about her husband, and she tells you that he is in the hospital. Mr. Smith started coughing up blood, so his wife took him to the hospital, where his PCP referred him to a cancer specialist. The pulmonary oncologist thinks that Mr. Smith may have bronchogenic carcinoma. Which test would the doctor order to examine lung secretions under a microscope to determine the presence of malignant cells?

   _____

(Continued)

8. Mr. Smith is confirmed to have cancer. The thoracic surgeon determines that there is a buildup of fluid in the pleural sac surrounding the affected lung. The surgeon schedules Mr. Smith for a procedure in which the fluid will be aspirated from this area. What is the term for this procedure?

_____

9. A week after this procedure is performed, the surgeon notices that fluid is continuing to build up in the area. This time, the surgeon recommends the placement of a chest tube that will drain the area. What is this procedure called?

_____

10. The surgeon orders a test to measure the amount of oxygen and carbon dioxide in Mr. Smith's blood. What is the name of this test?

_____

11. This test confirms that Mr. Smith's oxygen level is too low. What might the doctor order to help increase Mr. Smith's blood oxygen levels?

_____

12. You are enjoying a burger with your friends. You notice the man at the table next to you is eating and laughing loudly. Suddenly the man stops talking, puts his hands up to his throat, and tries to talk. You realize that this man's airway is obstructed and he is choking. What procedure must be performed on this man to clear his airway?

_____

13. You are outside mowing the lawn. You see your neighbor, Mr. Green, getting ready to run. Suddenly he falls to the ground. When you go to check on him, he is unresponsive. You notice that he is not breathing and does not have a heartbeat. You have been trained in an emergency lifesaving treatment that will attempt to restore normal cardiac and pulmonary functions. What is the name of this treatment?

_____

14. The emergency medical technicians arrive and take Mr. Green to the hospital in an ambulance. When you go to visit him later that day, you find out that the ER doctor put him on a machine that delivers artificial respirations because he is unable to breathe on his own. What is the name of this machine?

_____

15. To put Mr. Green on this machine, the ER doctor had to insert a breathing tube through his mouth and glottis, into the trachea. What is the name of this procedure?

_____

Preparing for Your Future in Healthcare

Match each of the following word parts with the correct meaning. You will not use all of the meanings.

_____ 1. cardi/o

_____ 2. pulmon/o

_____ 3. resuscit/o

_____ 4. spir/o

_____ 5. -centesis

_____ 6. -meter

_____ 7. -metry

_____ 8. -stomy

_____ 9. -tomy

A. breathing

B. surgical puncture to remove fluid

C. to revive

D. process of cutting; incision

E. heart

F. measure

G. surgical opening

H. narrowing; tightening

I. lung

J. process of measuring

Refer to the description of healthcare professionals on page 198 of your textbook. Then define the following terms. You may use the information in your textbook, a regular or medical dictionary, the glossary in the back of your textbook, and your own words to define the terms.

10. asthma: _____

_____

_____

_____

11. cerebral vascular accident: _____

_____

_____

_____

12. ventilator: _____

_____

_____

_____

13. thoracic cage: _____

_____

_____

_____

(Continued)

14. lobectomy: _____

_____

_____

_____

15. pulmonary function test: _____

_____

_____

_____

16. endotracheal intubation: _____

_____

_____

_____

Match the appropriate healthcare professional with each of the following descriptions or tasks. You will use each profession more than once.

A. respiratory therapist   C. pulmonologist
B. perfusionist   D. thoracic surgeon

_____ 17. requires a medical degree

_____ 18. may care for patients in their homes

_____ 19. performs surgery

_____ 20. part of the surgical team in the operating room for heart and lung surgeries

_____ 21. manages patients on ventilators

_____ 22. cares for patients in intensive care centers

_____ 23. manages the heart-lung machine

_____ 24. may work in a nursing home or long-term care facility

_____ 25. can administer blood products and medications

Name _____   Date _____

Chapter 7 Practice Test

Using the word parts on pages 175–176 and in Appendix A on pages 418–426 of your textbook, define the following medical terms.

1. rhinoplasty: _____

2. bronchoscopy: _____

3. laryngectomy: _____

4. hemoptysis: _____

Break down each medical term listed below by rewriting the term, and then placing a slash between each word part (prefix, root word, combining vowel, and suffix if used). Then define each term.

5. pneumonia

   Breakdown: _____

   Define: _____

6. pneumonomelanosis

   Breakdown: _____

   Define: _____

7. pneumonomycosis

   Breakdown: _____

   Define: _____

8. laryngalgia

   Breakdown: _____

   Define: _____

9. endotracheal

   Breakdown: _____

   Define: _____

10. bronchorrhaphy

    Breakdown: _____

    Define: _____

11. pleurodynia

    Breakdown: _____

    Define: _____

(Continued)

Name _____ Date _____

Answer the following questions.

12. Which gas is contained in the air that we breathe out?

_____

13. When taking a patient's vital signs, what is considered one respiration?

_____

14. What is considered a normal respiratory rate for a 16 y/o male?

_____

15. What substance makes up the larynx and enables the vocal cords to move and produce sound?

_____

Match each of the following breathing-related medical terms with the correct meaning. You will not use all of the meanings.

_____ 16. apnea

_____ 17. bradypnea

_____ 18. dyspnea

_____ 19. eupnea

_____ 20. hyperpnea

_____ 21. orthopnea

_____ 22. tachypnea

A. normal breathing
B. shallow breathing
C. fast breathing
D. without breathing
E. deep breathing
F. difficult breathing
G. straight breathing
H. slow breathing

Match each of the following diseases and conditions with the correct meaning. You will not use all of the meanings.

_____ 23. pleural effusion

_____ 24. empyema

_____ 25. hemothorax

_____ 26. croup

_____ 27. pulmonary embolism

_____ 28. cystic fibrosis

_____ 29. atelectasis

_____ 30. pharyngitis

A. a traveling blood clot that becomes lodged in a lung
B. childhood disease characterized by a "barking" cough
C. condition of a collapsed or airless lung
D. congenital disease that causes increased production of mucus in the lungs
E. the result of excessive fluid buildup in the pleural cavity
F. inflammation of the lungs caused by an infection or irritant
G. inflammation of the throat
H. the presence of pus in the pleural cavity
I. the presence of blood in the pleural cavity

The Digestive System

Name _____ Date _____

Understanding Word Parts

Match each of the following word parts with the correct meaning. You will not use all of the meanings.

_____ 1. enter/o

_____ 2. col/o

_____ 3. bil/i

_____ 4. gastr/o

_____ 5. inguin/o

_____ 6. gluc/o

_____ 7. lapar/o

_____ 8. proct/o

_____ 9. dent/i

_____ 10. cholecyst/o

A. abdominal wall; abdomen

B. gallbladder

C. gums

D. rectum; anus

E. stomach

F. sugar

G. bile; gall

H. intestines

I. tooth

J. colon; large intestine

K. groin

_____ 11. peri-

_____ 12. -chezia

_____ 13. pre-

_____ 14. -pepsia

_____ 15. dia-

_____ 16. -rrhea

_____ 17. -stomy

_____ 18. -orexia

_____ 19. -prandial

_____ 20. -emesis

A. vomiting

B. complete; through

C. surgical opening

D. before; in front of

E. abnormal condition

F. meal

G. defecation; elimination of wastes

H. flow; excessive discharge

I. appetite

J. around; surrounding

K. digestion

(Continued)

Name _____ Date _____

Use the following combining forms, prefixes, and suffixes listed on pages 204–206 of your textbook to build the medical term that corresponds to each of the following definitions.

21. Word part: col/o

    Definition: creation of a surgical opening in the colon

    Term: _____

22. Word part: lapar/o

    Definition: instrument used to view the abdomen

    Term: _____

23. Word part: an-

    Definition: condition of without an appetite

    Term: _____

24. Word part: -prandial

    Definition: after a meal

    Term: _____

Break down each of the following medical terms by rewriting the term, and then placing a slash between each word part (prefix, root word, combining vowel, and suffix if used). Then define each term.

25. gastroenteritis

    Breakdown: _____

    Define: _____

26. cholecystectomy

    Breakdown: _____

    Define: _____

27. oropharyngeal

    Breakdown: _____

    Define: _____

28. periodontist

    Breakdown: _____

    Define: _____

29. lithotripsy

    Breakdown: _____

    Define: _____

30. gingivectomy

    Breakdown: _____

    Define: _____

Interpreting Medical Records

Read the following medical records. Define the abbreviations and terms called out in each record, and then answer the questions that follow each medical record.

A. Notes from Dr. Orr, **ATT PHYS**, **GI** specialist to **RN**

Schedule **Pt** for an **OP EGD** and **colonoscopy**. Pt has **hx** of **GERD**. Remind Pt to be **n.p.o.** 12 hours prior to procedure.

---

1. ATT PHYS: _____

2. GI: _____

3. RN: _____

4. Pt: _____

5. OP: _____

6. EGD: _____

7. colonoscopy: _____

8. hx: _____

9. GERD: _____

10. n.p.o.: _____

11. Why do you think this patient is ordered to be n.p.o. prior to the procedure?

_____

_____

B. Notes from B. Kramer, Doctor of **Dental** Surgery to dental assistant

Set up appointment for Pt to see Dr. S. Adams, a specialist in **oral** surgery, to evaluate for possible **hemiglossectomy** because of oral cancer. Remind Pt to take his recent **CAT** scan films to the appointment. Instruct Pt that he will be discharged to home with a **NG** tube for nutritional support.

---

12. dental: _____

13. oral: _____

14. hemiglossectomy: _____

15. CAT: _____

16. NG: _____

17. Why do you think this patient will need the NG tube after surgery?

_____

_____

(Continued)

C. <u>Notes from T. Ayers</u>, **ER** <u>Physician Assistant, to pt's</u> **PCP**, <u>Dr. R. Bailey</u>

Pt was evaluated in ER with **c/o** chest tightness, **SOB** and **dyspepsia**. Pt was concerned that he was having an **MI**. **P** and **BP** were **WNL**. **Lab** test for **cardiac** enzymes and **EKG** to **R/O** MI was negative. **UGI** X-rays **Dx** a hiatal hernia. Instructed Pt to take **OTC** antacids **p.r.n.** 1 hour **p.c.** and at **hs**. Please follow up with pt for further **tx**.

18. ER: _____

19. PCP: _____

20. c/o: _____

21. SOB: _____

22. dyspepsia: _____

23. MI: _____

24. P: _____

25. BP: _____

26. WNL: _____

27. lab: _____

28. cardiac: _____

29. EKG: _____

30. R/O: _____

31. UGI: _____

32. Dx: _____

33. OTC: _____

34. p.r.n.: _____

35. p.c.: _____

36. hs: _____

37. tx: _____

38. Why might this patient have thought he was having an MI when he went into the ER?

_____

_____

_____

_____

Comprehending Anatomy and Physiology Terminology

Use a regular or medical dictionary, the glossary in the back of your textbook, and your own words to define the following terms.

1. ingestion: _____

2. absorption: _____

3. buccae: _____

4. gingiva: _____

5. deglutition: _____

Answer the following questions.

6. What is the function of bile?

_____

_____

_____

7. What makes it possible for some medications to be absorbed under the tongue?

_____

_____

_____

8. What is the function of the enzyme you named in the previous question?

_____

_____

_____

9. Which term describes the ring-like muscle at the end of the esophagus that controls the flow of substances?

_____

10. Which term describes the upper part of the stomach?

_____

(Continued)

Name _____   Date _____

Match each of the following terms, which are related to a part of the intestine, with the correct meaning. You will not use all of the meanings.

_____ 11. duodenum

_____ 12. jejunum

_____ 13. ileum

_____ 14. cecum

_____ 15. appendix

_____ 16. ascending colon

_____ 17. transverse colon

_____ 18. descending colon

_____ 19. sigmoid colon

_____ 20. rectum

A. pouch that connects to the distal end of the ileum

B. section of the large intestine that starts at the cecum and ends below the liver

C. 12-foot section of the small intestine where vitamin B_{12} is absorbed

D. part of the large intestine that is named because of its shape

E. first section of the small intestine, where absorption of nutrients begins

F. section of the large intestine that starts on the left lateral side of the body and ends in the left inferior portion of the abdominal cavity

G. the middle section of the small intestine, which measures about 8 feet in length

H. storage area for feces

I. last section of the digestive tract, where feces are expelled from the body

J. appendage of the cecum that has no known function

K. the longest section of the large intestine

Label the different sections of the large intestine in the following image.

21. _____

22. _____

23. _____

24. _____

25. _____

26. _____

27. _____

28. _____

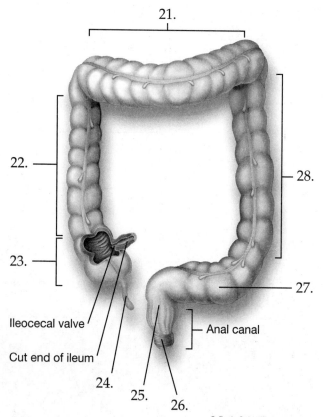

Ileocecal valve

Cut end of ileum

Anal canal

© Body Scientific International

Understanding Terms Related to Diseases and Conditions

Using the information on pages 204–206 of your textbook, define the following word parts.

1. -orexia: _____

2. appendic/o: _____

3. chol/e: _____

4. cirrh/o: _____

5. dent/i: _____

6. hepat/o: _____

7. inguin/o: _____

8. pancreat/o: _____

9. odont/o: _____

Match each of the following medical terms with the correct meaning. You will not use all of the meanings.

_____ 10. gastroenteritis

_____ 11. volvulus

_____ 12. anorexia nervosa

_____ 13. cholelithiasis

_____ 14. peritonitis

_____ 15. dental caries

_____ 16. esophageal varices

_____ 17. hiatal hernia

_____ 18. ulcerative colitis

_____ 19. hepatitis

_____ 20. cirrhosis

_____ 21. appendicitis

A. condition in which the upper part of the stomach protrudes through the esophageal opening in the diaphragm

B. condition in which the muscular motion of the intestines stops

C. condition involving self-deprivation of food and pathological weight loss

D. inflammation of the abdominal cavity

E. tooth decay that leads to cavities

F. the presence of stones in the gallbladder

G. inflammation of the appendix

H. inflammation of the liver, generally caused by a viral infection

I. scarring of the liver, generally caused by alcohol and/or drug abuse or chronic liver inflammation

J. chronic inflammation of the colon with ulcers

K. abnormal twisting of the intestines

L. swollen, twisted veins in the lower end of the esophagus

M. inflammation of the stomach and small intestines

(Continued)

Name _____ Date _____

Choose the correct term for each sign or symptom of a GI disorder.

_____ 22. vomiting blood
     A. hemoptysis   C. hematemesis
     B. hematochezia   D. hemorrhage

_____ 23. painful or difficult swallowing
     A. dysphonia   C. dyspepsia
     B. dysphagia   D. dyspnea

_____ 24. abnormal accumulation of fluid in the abdomen
     A. constipation   C. diarrhea
     B. cirrhosis   D. ascites

_____ 25. yellow discoloration of the skin due to blood disorder
     A. cyanosis   C. jaundice
     B. cirrhosis   D. peritonitis

_____ 26. bad breath
     A. flatus   C. jaundice
     B. eructation   D. halitosis

_____ 27. unpleasant sensation in the stomach that causes an urge to vomit
     A. anorexia   C. emesis
     B. nausea   D. dyspepsia

_____ 28. the backwards flow of food into the esophagus
     A. regurgitation   C. dysphagia
     B. dyspepsia   D. borborygmus

_____ 29. lack of appetite
     A. nausea   C. regurgitation
     B. emesis   D. anorexia

_____ 30. movement of gas in the digestive tract that makes rumbling sounds in the abdomen
     A. borborygmus   C. regurgitation
     B. flatus   D. emesis

Name _____ Date _____

Analyzing Diagnostic- and Treatment-Related Terms

Read the following scenarios and answer the question in each one.

1. Mr. Barker is a 51 y/o male. His father died at age 68 of colon cancer. Mr. Barker's PCP performed an office procedure in which only the sigmoid colon was examined using a scope. What is the name of this test?

   _____

2. Mr. Barker's PCP referred him to a GI specialist, Dr. Miller, to be evaluated for colon cancer. Dr. Miller recommended that Mr. Barker undergo a test to visually examine the colon with a scope. What is the name of this test?

   _____

3. During the procedure, Dr. Miller noticed a colon polyp in the distal end of the descending colon. The doctor removed the entire polyp and gave it to the nurse to be evaluated under a microscope to see if it is cancerous. What is the name of this test?

   _____

4. Dr. Miller decided to order further testing on Mr. Barker. He ordered a test in which barium (a contrast agent) is put into the rectum and X-rays are taken of the lower part of the digestive tract. What is the name of this test?

   _____

5. Mr. Rodriguez is a 62 y/o male who noticed some bright red blood in the toilet after going to the bathroom. He contacted his PCP, Dr. Pena. Which term might Mr. Rodriguez use to describe this symptom?

   _____

6. Before Mr. Rodriguez came into the office, Dr. Pena wanted him to take a sample of his feces to the laboratory. At the laboratory, healthcare professionals evaluated the sample to see if there is any blood present. What is the name of this test?

   _____

7. Dr. Pena had Mr. Rodriguez come into the office so he could perform a visual examination of the rectum using a scope. What is the name of this test?

   _____

8. Mrs. Thomas visited the radiology department of the hospital, where she was scheduled to have a test that uses sound waves to generate an image of the abdominal organs. During this test, healthcare professionals will check her gallbladder to see if stones are present. What is the name of this test?

   _____

9. If there are stones in Mrs. Thomas' gallbladder, what term would a healthcare professional use to describe her condition?

   _____

(Continued)

10. Miss Davis has been experiencing stomach pain for several months. Her doctor ordered a blood test to see if she has the bacteria known as *H. pylori* in her body. What is the name of this test?

_____

11. Mr. Stevens has been having problems swallowing. His doctor ordered a test in which Mr. Stevens drinks a substance that will show up on a specialized X-ray. Pictures are taken while Mr. Stevens is swallowing the substance so that the doctor can evaluate his swallowing mechanism. What is the name of this test?

_____

12. Which medical term describes the problem that Mr. Stevens is experiencing?

_____

13. Clare is a nurse practitioner in an outpatient drug and alcohol treatment center. One of the patients she cares for has been complaining of right upper abdominal pain. Clare is concerned that this patient may have a condition that involves scarring of the liver. She ordered a blood test that will measure the different enzymes used in the function of the liver. What is the name of this test?

_____

14. Which term describes the medical condition that Clare suspects this patient has?

_____

15. Deidre is a 45 y/o female with complaints of epigastric pain. A physician assistant in the clinic referred her to a GI specialist to have several tests performed. One of the tests will take place in the radiology department of the hospital. Deidre will be given barium to drink, and then X-rays of her stomach and duodenum will be taken. What is the name of this test?

_____

16. Deidre is also scheduled to have a test performed in which the GI specialist will put a fiber-optic scope in her mouth, down the esophagus, to the stomach, and into the duodenum. What is the name of this test?

_____

17. Describe where Deidre's *epigastric* pain is located.

_____

18. Chloe is a 16 y/o female who has been receiving chemotherapy treatment for leukemia. She has been experiencing some side effects of the treatment, including anorexia and hyperemesis. Describe what the term *hyperemesis* means.

_____

19. What type of medication might the doctor give Chloe to help relieve her hyperemesis?

_____

20. Heather is a 26 y/o who has had problems with weight management since she was in high school. She has tried dieting and exercise but has been unable to lose weight. She is considering having surgery that will reduce the size of her stomach. What is this type of surgery called?

_____

Preparing for Your Future in Healthcare

Match the appropriate healthcare professional with each of the following scenarios. You will use each profession more than once.

dental hygienist   dentist   gastroenterologist   registered dietitian

1. A professional model who noticed a stain on her front tooth contacts this healthcare professional to have the stain removed.

   _____

2. A 42 y/o male with pain and swelling in his left lower jaw for three days saw his primary care physician, who said he has an abscessed (infected) tooth that may need to be pulled. The PCP refers her patient to this healthcare professional.

   _____

3. A 25 y/o pregnant female has been diagnosed with gestational diabetes. Her OB/GYN wants her to meet with this healthcare professional to help develop a diet plan to follow during her pregnancy.

   _____

4. A 23 y/o female college student has been experiencing diarrhea for several days, followed by constipation. She also reports bloating, abdominal cramping, and weight loss. The nurse practitioner (NP) who has been seeing this patient is concerned that she has irritable bowel syndrome. The NP will refer her to this specialist for treatment options.

   _____

5. A 12 y/o male has a fractured tooth after being hit in the face with a softball. His mom calls this healthcare professional to make an appointment for him.

   _____

6. A 54 y/o high school teacher needs to make his six-month follow-up appointment for a teeth cleaning. He would make an appointment with this healthcare professional.

   _____

7. A 45 y/o female comes into the local food pantry asking for help with meal planning. Her daughter was recently diagnosed with celiac disease, and she doesn't understand what kinds of foods her daughter should avoid. She is scared that her daughter will get sick again. The counselors at the food pantry would recommend the woman see this healthcare professional.

   _____

8. An 80 y/o female resident of a nursing home has not had a bowel movement in five days. When the resident says she needs to use the toilet, the nurse aide assists her. After the aide helps the resident back into her wheelchair, the aide notices bright red blood in the toilet. The aide reports this to his charge nurse. The charge nurse documents the occurrence of constipation and hematochezia in the resident's chart. The charge nurse would make an appointment with this healthcare professional for the resident.

   _____

Name _____   Date _____

Chapter 8 Practice Test

Using the word parts on pages 204–206 of your textbook, define the following medical terms.

1. hyperemesis: _____

2. hepatorrhaphy: _____

3. cholecystalgia: _____

4. dentalgia: _____

5. nasogastric: _____

Break down each medical term listed below by rewriting the term, and then placing a slash between each word part (prefix, root word, combining vowel, and suffix if used). Then define each term.

6. abdominocentesis

   Breakdown: _____

   Define: _____

7. colostomy

   Breakdown: _____

   Define: _____

8. hepatocyte

   Breakdown: _____

   Define: _____

9. pharyngoplasty

   Breakdown: _____

   Define: _____

10. splenorrhaphy

    Breakdown: _____

    Define: _____

11. proctosigmoidoscopy

    Breakdown: _____

    Define: _____

(Continued)

Name _____ Date _____

Answer the following questions.

12. Which type of digestion involves saliva secreted by the salivary glands?

_____

13. What is the purpose of the uvula?

_____

14. Which term describes the mixture of partially digested food and gastric juices that passes from the stomach into the first section of the small intestine?

_____

15. What is the largest internal organ in the body?

_____

Identify the term that corresponds to each disease or condition described below.

16. a chronic disease that causes inflammation of the digestive tract and generally affects the ileum

    and the colon: _____

17. the chronic viral infection that causes liver inflammation and damage and is usually transmitted

    by blood or body fluids during sexual contact or childbirth: _____

18. the condition that occurs due to high levels of bilirubin in the blood: _____

Match each of the following terms with the correct meaning. You will not use all of the meanings.

_____ 19. proctoscopy	A. surgical procedure in which a portion of the colon is diverted to an artificial opening in the abdominal wall
_____ 20. antiemetic	B. drug used to stimulate defecation
_____ 21. barium enema	C. test that detects the presence of hidden blood in the feces
_____ 22. EGD	D. visual examination of the large intestines using a scope
_____ 23. colonoscopy	E. laboratory test that detects the presence of pathogens in the blood
_____ 24. capsule endoscopy	F. laboratory test that measures the number and types of cells in the blood
_____ 25. laxative	G. visual examination of the esophagus, stomach, and first part of the small intestines using a scope
_____ 26. occult blood test	H. visual examination of the rectum using a scope
_____ 27. serology test	I. visual examination of the digestive tract using a wireless camera
_____ 28. bariatric surgery	J. X-ray of the large intestine and rectum using a contrast medium
_____ 29. CBC	K. laboratory test that measures the amount of pancreatic enzymes in the blood
_____ 30. colostomy	L. drug that prevents or relieves nausea and vomiting
	M. surgical procedure used to treat morbid obesity

Chapter 9

The Nervous System

Name _____   Date _____

Understanding Word Parts

Match each of the following word parts with the correct meaning. You will not use all of the meanings.

_____ 1. -paresis

_____ 2. -sclerosis

_____ 3. -rrhaphy

_____ 4. -phasia

_____ 5. -algesia

_____ 6. -cele

_____ 7. -plegia

_____ 8. -leptic

_____ 9. con-

_____ 10. sub-

A. hernia; swelling; protrusion

B. speech

C. to seize; take hold of

D. below; under

E. suture

F. pertaining to blood condition

G. weakness

H. pain; sensitivity

I. hardening; thickening

J. paralysis

K. together; with

_____ 11. schiz/o

_____ 12. poli/o

_____ 13. hydr/o

_____ 14. radicul/o

_____ 15. troph/o

_____ 16. encephal/o

_____ 17. cephal/o

_____ 18. phas/o

_____ 19. tax/o

_____ 20. gli/o

A. speech

B. brain

C. extreme

D. glue

E. head

F. gray matter

G. nerve root

H. development; nourishment

I. split

J. coordination; order

K. water

(Continued)

Name _____ Date _____

Use the following prefixes and suffixes listed on pages 237–239 of your textbook to build the medical term that corresponds to each of the following definitions.

21. Word part: -al

    Definition: pertaining to fainting

    Term: _____

22. Word part: -algia

    Definition: nerve pain

    Term: _____

23. Word part: -ia

    Definition: condition of faulty or difficult speech

    Term: _____

24. Word part: -ia

    Definition: condition of difficulty with words

    Term: _____

25. Word part: -algia

    Definition: head pain (headache)

    Term: _____

26. Word part: an-

    Definition: without feeling or sensation

    Term: _____

Break down each of the following medical terms by rewriting the term, and then placing a slash between each word part (prefix, root word, combining vowel, and suffix if used). Then define each term.

27. schizophrenia

    Breakdown: _____

    Define: _____

28. hydrocephalus

    Breakdown: _____

    Define: _____

29. meningocele

    Breakdown: _____

    Define: _____

30. ischemia

    Breakdown: _____

    Define: _____

Interpreting Medical Records

Read the following medical records. Define the abbreviations and terms called out in each record, and then answer the questions that follow each medical record.

> 20 y/o female college student with **PMH** of mild **CP** presents to on-campus medical clinic with **c/o** severe **HA**, fever, fatigue, and **photophobia**. Pt has a positive Babinski sign. Clinic physician assistant has ordered **LP** to collect and analyze sample of **CSF** to **R/O** bacterial **meningitis**.

1. PMH: _____

2. CP: _____

3. c/o: _____

4. HA: _____

5. photophobia: _____

_____

_____

6. LP: _____

7. CSF: _____

8. R/O: _____

9. meningitis: _____

_____

_____

10. What is the Babinski sign?

_____

_____

_____

_____

_____

_____

_____

(Continued)

72 y/o male admitted to **ER** by ambulance with c/o **dystaxia**, numbness on the **L** side of his face and arm, **dysphasia**, and **dysphagia**. Pt's wife states that he seemed to "black out" for about 30 seconds, and then fell onto the bed. She also stated that Pt saw his **PCP** last week and was **Dx** with **TIA**.

PE: left sided weakness noted

Plan: **MRI** head **STAT** to **R/O CVA**

11. ER: _____

12. dystaxia: _____

_____

_____

13. L: _____

14. dysphasia: _____

_____

_____

15. dysphagia: _____

_____

_____

16. PCP: _____

17. Dx: _____

18. TIA: _____

19. PE: _____

20. MRI: _____

21. STAT: _____

22. R/O: _____

23. CVA: _____

24. Why was the Dx of TIA important in this case?

_____

_____

_____

_____

_____

(Continued)

24 y/o male was transported to ER after being involved in a motorcycle accident. Pt was not wearing a helmet. **CT** shows **SDH**. MRI reveals **SCI**. Admitted to critical care unit to perform **EEG** and monitor **ICP**.

25. CT: _____

26. SDH: _____

27. SCI: _____

28. EEG: _____

29. ICP: _____

30. Explain where a SDH might be located.

_____

_____

_____

_____

10 y/o male was referred by pediatrician to child psychiatry for evaluation due to poor grades and difficulty sitting in class. Pt's mother reports that pt has been getting into trouble at school. Pt's mother also reports that she and Pt's dad have recently divorced. Mental health specialist Dx Pt with **ADHD** and **GAD**. Recommends Pt undergo **OP CBT**.

31. ADHD: _____

32. GAD: _____

33. OP: _____

34. CBT: _____

35. What may be one cause of the Pt's GAD?

_____

_____

_____

_____

Comprehending Anatomy and Physiology Terminology

Use a regular or medical dictionary, the glossary in the back of your textbook, and your own words to define the following terms.

1. homeostasis: _____

   _____

2. neurons: _____

   _____

3. neuroglial cells: _____

   _____

4. sensory neurons: _____

   _____

5. motor neurons: _____

   _____

6. central nervous system: _____

   _____

7. peripheral nervous system: _____

   _____

8. reflex: _____

   _____

9. autonomic nervous system: _____

   _____

10. somatic nervous system: _____

    _____

11. sympathetic nervous system: _____

    _____

12. parasympathetic nervous system: _____

    _____

(Continued)

Answer the following questions.

13. Which body system does the nervous system work closely with to help maintain homeostasis?

_____

14. Which term describes changes in the internal or external environments that can cause a nervous system response?

_____

15. What is the process by which the central nervous system interprets all the information it receives from organs such as the eyes and the skin?

_____

16. Which division of the nervous system makes voluntary movement possible?

_____

17. Which term describes the process of transmitting nerve impulses from the brain and spinal cord to all other parts of the body?

_____

18. What is the difference between gray matter and white matter?

_____

19. Which term describes the connective tissues that surround the CNS?

_____

Match each of the following terms related to the brain with the correct meaning. You will not use all of the meanings.

_____ 20. cerebrum

_____ 21. gyri

_____ 22. corpus callosum

_____ 23. frontal lobe

_____ 24. parietal lobe

_____ 25. temporal lobe

_____ 26. cerebellum

_____ 27. diencephalon

_____ 28. hypothalamus

_____ 29. pineal gland

_____ 30. brain stem

A. area of the brain that processes stimuli related to touch and pain

B. convolutions on the surface of the brain

C. part of the brain that controls balance and equilibrium

D. serves as the conduit for sensory information between the cerebrum or cerebellum and the rest of the body

E. the largest region of the brain

F. substance that protects the brain and spinal cord from injury

G. area of the brain that controls language processing

H. the connection between the left and right hemispheres of the brain

I. area of the brain that controls hunger, thirst, and digestion

J. area of the brain that is the "seat of your personality"

K. the site of three key glands

L. gland that secretes melatonin

Understanding Terms Related to Diseases and Conditions

Match each of the following terms related to neurological conditions with the correct meaning. You will not use all of the meanings.

_____ 1. aura

_____ 2. coma

_____ 3. concussion

_____ 4. convulsion

_____ 5. delirium

_____ 6. dementia

_____ 7. headache

_____ 8. hemiplegia

_____ 9. paralysis

_____ 10. paraplegia

_____ 11. paresthesia

_____ 12. seizure

_____ 13. syncope

_____ 14. tremor

A. state of mental confusion, agitation, and disorientation

B. paralysis of the lower half of the body

C. loss of voluntary motor function

D. traumatic brain injury due to a blow to the head or violent shaking of the body

E. involuntary trembling or shaking of the body or limbs

F. disruption of the electrical activity of the brain

G. progressive mental deterioration caused by organic brain disease

H. a sensation that often occurs before a seizure or migraine

I. sensation of numbness, prickling, or tingling

J. diffuse pain in one or more parts of the head

K. a state of extended unconsciousness

L. a sudden, abnormal, involuntary contraction of the muscles

M. unilateral paralysis of the face

N. fainting

O. paralysis of one side of the body

Read the following scenarios and answer the question in each one.

15. A 17-year-old linebacker for the high school football team had a helmet-to-helmet collision with the running back from the opposing team. The linebacker was assisted off the field and evaluated by the trainer, who recommended that he be evaluated in the emergency room. The MRI in the emergency room showed bruising of the cerebral tissue. What is the diagnosis for this patient?

_____

16. An abdominal ultrasound of a pregnant woman shows that her baby has a protrusion of the spinal cord and meninges. What is the baby's diagnosis?

_____

17. A 68-year-old man comes to the hospital because his wife has noticed he's having trouble holding things. He also walks slowly and has a difficult time walking in the store with his wife. When the doctor examines this man, she notices that his posture is more stooped than the last time he was examined, about six months earlier. What is the patient's diagnosis?

_____

(Continued)

18. A 43-year-old female was discharged from the hospital after spending almost two weeks there due to a severe respiratory viral infection. One week later, she returned to the emergency room with complaints of muscle pain and weakness that had gotten progressively worse since she was discharged from the hospital. She had also noticed that she lost voluntary movement of her fingers. What is this patient's diagnosis?

_____

19. A 5-year-old male was admitted to the pediatric intensive care unit by his pediatrician because he developed symptoms of confusion and didn't know who his mother was. He had two seizures on the way to the doctor's office and became unconscious. The pediatric neurologist also noticed that this patient has hepatomegaly. What is the patient's diagnosis?

_____

Choose the correct mental health disorder for each of the following descriptions.

_____ 20. This developmental disability appears in childhood, and it is characterized by difficulty communicating and making eye contact with others, as well as repetitive motor activities, such as rocking back and forth.
   A. ADHD   C. ASD
   B. dyslexia   D. ID

_____ 21. In this mental disorder, a person will eat large amounts of food, and then purge through induced vomiting or use of laxatives. Excessive exercise may also occur.
   A. anorexia nervosa   C. seasonal affective disorder
   B. schizophrenia   D. bulimia nervosa

_____ 22. This mood disorder is characterized by severe sadness and lack of interest in normal activities. Symptoms generally occur around the winter months.
   A. SAD   C. postpartum psychosis
   B. bipolar disorder   D. OCD

_____ 23. In this anxiety disorder, a person will perform the same activity over and over, such as washing his or her hands every hour even though the skin is dry, cracked, and extremely painful.
   A. panic disorder   C. PTSD
   B. GAD
   D. OCD

_____ 24. This mental disorder is commonly seen in soldiers who return from war. These soldiers may experience exaggerated fears and difficulty sleeping.
   A. PD   C. OCD
   B. PTSD   D. GAD

_____ 25. In this mental disorder, a person may be abnormally happy one day and so extremely sad the next day that he or she cannot get out of bed.
   A. SAD   C. bipolar disorder
   B. postpartum psychosis   D. schizophrenia

Analyzing Diagnostic- and Treatment-Related Terms

Using the word parts on pages 237–239 of your textbook, define the following medical terms.

1. ischemia: _____

   _____

2. neuroleptic: _____

   _____

3. hypnotic: _____

   _____

4. anesthetic: _____

   _____

5. subdural: _____

   _____

6. anxiolytic: _____

   _____

7. myelogram: _____

   _____

8. craniectomy: _____

   _____

Identify the term that corresponds to each diagnostic test or treatment method described below.

9. measures the speed at which electrical impulses travel through a nerve and can be used to diagnose carpal tunnel syndrome or myasthenia gravis:

   _____

10. a record of the electrical impulses of the brain; useful in evaluating seizure disorders, strokes, and the brain function of coma patients:

   _____

11. X-ray of the spinal cord that is useful in evaluating spinal tumors, herniated vertebral disks, or spinal stenosis: _____

12. test in which the reflexes on the plantar surface of the foot are stimulated to assist in diagnosing neurological disorders such as brain tumors and meningitis:

   _____

(Continued)

13. two tests that can be performed to assist in diagnosing a CVA:

   _____

14. test that involves collecting and evaluating CSF and can assist in diagnosing meningitis, Guillain-Barré syndrome, or cancers of the brain and spinal cord:

   _____

15. pain management procedure in which an anesthetic is injected into an area near a nerve:

   _____

16. surgical repair of a nerve:

   _____

17. surgical procedure in which the inner layer of a carotid artery is cleared of fatty plaque deposits to improve blood flow to the brain:

   _____

18. surgical procedure that treats a herniated disk of the spine, in which all or part of the lamina of a vertebra is removed:

   _____

19. procedure used to treat severe depression, in which electrical shocks are applied to the brain:

   _____

Match each of the following types of drugs with the correct meaning.

_____ 20. sedative

_____ 21. analgesic

_____ 22. anticonvulsant

_____ 23. hypnotic

_____ 24. anesthetic

_____ 25. anxiolytic

A. causes a loss of sensation

B. reduces feelings of anxiety

C. promotes sleep and loss of consciousness

D. relieves pain

E. produces a soothing or tranquilizing effect

F. treats convulsions

Preparing for Your Future in Healthcare

Use the information on pages 237–239 of your textbook to define the following word parts.

1. crani/o: _____

2. dur/a: _____

3. encephal/o: _____

4. hypn/o: _____

5. neur/o: _____

6. psych/o: _____

7. traumat/o: _____

8. -esthesia: _____

9. -tomy: _____

10. -ectomy: _____

11. -ist: _____

12. -pathy: _____

Use a regular or medical dictionary, the glossary in the back of your textbook, and your own words to define the following terms.

13. electroneurodiagnostic technician: _____

_____

_____

14. anesthetic: _____

_____

_____

15. hypnotic: _____

_____

_____

16. sedative: _____

_____

_____

(Continued)

Name _____ Date _____

17. neuropathy: _____

_____

_____

18. epilepsy: _____

_____

_____

19. cerebrovascular accident: _____

_____

_____

20. aneurysm: _____

_____

_____

21. Parkinson's disease: _____

_____

_____

Match the appropriate healthcare professional with each of the following descriptions or tasks. You will use each profession more than once.

    A. anesthesiologist   B. electroneurodiagnostic   C. neurosurgeon
                                            technician

_____ 22. requires a medical degree

_____ 23. may work in a sleep disorder lab

_____ 24. may perform a craniotomy

_____ 25. closely monitors a patient's heart rate

_____ 26. requires a doctor's order to perform any test

_____ 27. works in an operating room

_____ 28. may repair an aneurysm

_____ 29. administers drugs

_____ 30. may perform an EEG

Chapter 9 Practice Test

Using the word parts on pages 237–239 and 418–426 of your textbook, identify the medical term that corresponds to each of the following definitions.

1. inflammation of the brain: _____

2. inflammation of the brain and spinal cord: _____

3. inflammation of the membranes around the brain and spinal cord: _____

4. paralysis of all four extremities: _____

5. disease of a nerve: _____

Break down each medical term listed below by rewriting the term, and then placing a slash between each word part (prefix, root word, combining vowel, and suffix if used). Then define each term.

6. encephalomyelopathy

   Breakdown: _____

   Define: _____

7. anesthesiologist

   Breakdown: _____

   Define: _____

8. radiculopathy

   Breakdown: _____

   Define: _____

9. hydrocephalus

   Breakdown: _____

   Define: _____

10. causalgia

    Breakdown: _____

    Define: _____

11. aphasia

    Breakdown: _____

    Define: _____

12. anencephaly

    Breakdown: _____

    Define: _____

(Continued)

Name _____ Date _____

13. neuroma

    Breakdown: _____

    Define: _____

14. poliomyelitis

    Breakdown: _____

    Define: _____

15. cerebrovascular

    Breakdown: _____

    Define: _____

Label the different parts of the brain in the following image.

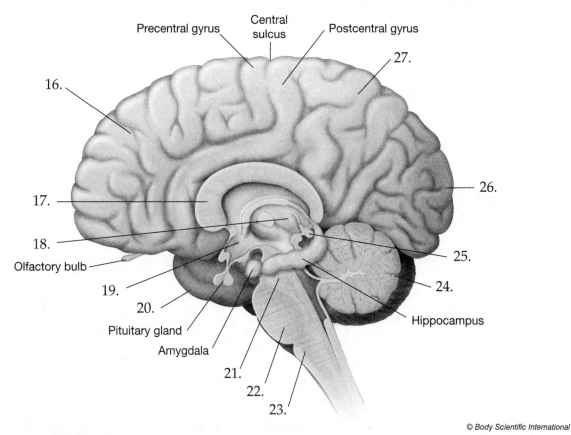

© Body Scientific International

16. _____   22. _____

17. _____   23. _____

18. _____   24. _____

19. _____   25. _____

20. _____   26. _____

21. _____   27. _____

(Continued)

Name _____ Date _____

Match each of the following medical terms or abbreviations with the correct meaning. You will not use all of the meanings.

_____ 28. ALS

_____ 29. Bell's palsy

_____ 30. cerebral aneurysm

_____ 31. CP

_____ 32. CVA

_____ 33. concussion

_____ 34. delirium

_____ 35. dementia

_____ 36. epilepsy

_____ 37. GB syndrome

_____ 38. MS

_____ 39. MG

_____ 40. hydrocephalus

_____ 41. meningocele

_____ 42. myelomeningocele

_____ 43. polio

_____ 44. grand mal seizure

_____ 45. TIA

A. condition in which neuromuscular communication is disrupted and the muscles become severely weakened

B. a disruption of electrical activity in the brain characterized by violent muscle contractions and loss of consciousness

C. a state of confusion, agitation, and disorientation, usually accompanied by hallucinations

D. a condition that occurs at or before birth, which affects movement and muscle tone

E. the generalized term that describes the neurological disorder in which cells in the brain do not function correctly, causing seizures

F. accumulation of CSF in the ventricles of the brain, which results in cephalomegaly and may cause brain damage

G. abnormal, localized dilation of a blood vessel in the cerebrum

H. a condition in which a newborn baby's meninges protrude through an opening of the skull or spinal cord

I. a TBI resulting from a blow to the head or severe shaking of the head and upper body

J. inflammation of multiple peripheral nerves, causing progressive muscle weakness

K. condition caused by the degeneration of motor neurons in the spinal cord and in the brain's medulla and cortex

L. condition generally discovered in newborns, in which a portion of the spinal cord and meninges protrudes through an opening in the spine

M. condition characterized by unilateral facial paralysis

N. condition caused by organic brain disease, which is characterized by memory loss, dysphonia, and difficulty performing routine tasks

O. a brief stoppage of blood flow to a part of the brain

P. inflammation of the gray matter of the spinal cord

Q. occurrence of a painful rash, generally on the torso which is caused by the varicella-zoster virus

R. the sudden blockage of blood flow to the brain that results in death of brain tissue

S. chronic, slow-progressing disease characterized by dyskinesia, dystaxia, paresthesia, and muscle weakness

The Special Senses

Name _____ Date _____

Understanding Word Parts

Match each of the following word parts with the correct meaning. You will not use all of the meanings.

_____ 1. exo-

_____ 2. -ous

_____ 3. -cusis

_____ 4. -metry

_____ 5. -opia

_____ 6. -itis

_____ 7. eso-

_____ 8. -oma

_____ 9. -ptosis

_____ 10. hypo-

_____ 11. -tropia

_____ 12. -osmia

_____ 13. a-

_____ 14. -pathy

_____ 15. -otia

A. within; into

B. droop; sag; prolapse; protrude

C. ear condition

D. disease

E. to turn

F. smell condition

G. not; without

H. outward

I. inflammation

J. hearing

K. tumor; mass

L. pertaining to

M. vision condition

N. below; below normal; deficient

O. process of measuring

P. inward

(Continued)

_____ 16. presby/o

_____ 17. dacry/o

_____ 18. gustat/o

_____ 19. mydr/o

_____ 20. phak/o

_____ 21. blephar/o

_____ 22. phot/o

_____ 23. dipl/o

_____ 24. nyct/o

_____ 25. core/o

_____ 26. glauc/o

_____ 27. salping/o

_____ 28. myring/o

_____ 29. scot/o

_____ 30. ocul/o

A. gray

B. auditory tube; fallopian tube

C. pupil

D. eye

E. double

F. sebum; fat

G. night

H. light

I. eardrum

J. eyelid

K. darkness

L. widened; enlarged

M. old age

N. lens of the eye

O. tear

P. taste

Use the following prefixes, combining forms, and suffixes listed on pages 275–276 of your textbook to build the medical term that corresponds to each of the following definitions.

31. Word part: an-

    Definition: condition of having no smell sense

    Term: _____

32. Word part: audi/o

    Definition: process of measuring hearing

    Term: _____

33. Word part: -algia

    Definition: ear pain

    Term: _____

34. Word part: -tic

    Definition: pertaining to (making) smaller

    Term: _____

(Continued)

Break down each of the following medical terms by rewriting the term, and then placing a slash between each word part (prefix, root word, combining vowel, and suffix if used). Then define each term.

35. dacryocystitis

    Breakdown: _____

    Define: _____

36. amblyopia

    Breakdown: _____

    Define: _____

37. myringoplasty

    Breakdown: _____

    Define: _____

38. retinoscope

    Breakdown: _____

    Define: _____

39. otosclerosis

    Breakdown: _____

    Define: _____

40. lacrimal

    Breakdown: _____

    Define: _____

Interpreting Medical Records

Read the following medical record. Define the abbreviations and terms called out in the record, and then answer the question that follows.

<u>See Clearly Eye Clinic</u>

<u>Dr. Ken U. Seamy</u>

Patient Name: Jose Ramirez

Date of Exam: April 3, 2017

Medical Record No.: R3456

CC: **Pt c/o** difficulty with nighttime driving. Pt states, "I see halos around the lights when I try to drive after dusk." Pt states that this has restricted his activity, and that he must leave work early to avoid driving at night.

HPI: 62 y/o Hispanic male presents to clinic with c/o decreased **VA**, both distance and close up. He also states that his vision seems more "dull and cloudy" than normal. He first noticed symptoms about six month ago, and the visual problems have worsened since then. Pt currently does not wear glasses, but he states that he is "afraid that I am going to have to start wearing them because when I read the newspaper the words are blurry."

PMH: **HTN** controlled with diet and medication.

SH: **Hx** of smoking, but Pt states he quit about five years ago when he experienced an episode of **angina** and was **Dx** with **CAD**.

OH: Retired from the Army. Currently works as supervisor for a building construction company.

Current Medications: **OTC** multivitamins, fish oil. Prescription medications include lisinopril 20 **mg b.i.d.**, Lipitor 20 mg once a day.

PE: **BP**: 136/78. **PERRLA**, brows symmetrical, lashes intact, conjunctiva pink, no discharge noted, sclera white. VA 20/40 on **Snellen chart**. VA 20/30 with corrective lenses. VA 20/60 with glare test. **Bilateral** nuclear sclerotic cataracts noted.

Plan: Bilateral **phaco** with IOL (intraocular lens) implants. Schedule **O.D.** first, and then plan for second procedure on **O.S.** two weeks after that. Inform Pt that he will be able to return to work two days **postop**, but he should not lift anything over 10 pounds and needs to restrict outdoor exposure from two days **preop** to two weeks postop.

Medications to Be Dispensed:

Gaifloxacin ophthalmic solution: 4 **gtts q.i.d.** O.D. two days preop until two weeks postop

Ketoralac NSAID solution: 1 gtt every day two days preop until two weeks postop

Prednisolone ophthalmic solution: 1 gtt **t.i.d.** two days preop until one week postop

Repeat this order for O.S.

(Continued)

Name _____ Date _____

1. CC: _____

2. Pt: _____

3. c/o: _____

4. HPI: _____

5. VA: _____

6. PMH: _____

7. HTN: _____

8. SH: _____

9. Hx: _____

10. angina: _____

11. Dx: _____

12. CAD: _____

13. OH: _____

14. OTC: _____

15. mg: _____

16. b.i.d.: _____

17. PE: _____

18. BP: _____

19. PERRLA: _____

20. Snellen chart: _____

21. bilateral: _____

22. phaco: _____

23. O.D.: _____

24. O.S.: _____

25. postop: _____

26. preop: _____

27. gtt: _____

28. q.i.d.: _____

29. t.i.d.: _____

30. Which medical term describes the visual condition that this patient experiences when he is reading the newspaper?

_____

Comprehending Anatomy and Physiology Terminology

Use pages 277–284 and the glossary in the back of your textbook to define the following terms.

1. accommodation: _____

2. blind spot: _____

3. visual acuity: _____

4. pinna: _____

5. umami: _____

Answer the following questions.

6. What is the general function of the eyes, ears, nose, tongue, and skin—collectively known as the *specialized sense organs*?

   _____

7. Which term describes the "white of the eye"?

   _____

8. What is the purpose of the cornea?

   _____

9. Describe the ciliary muscle's function.

   _____

10. What substance is located in the front chamber of the eyeball?

    _____

11. What substance is located in the back chamber of the eyeball?

    _____

12. Which structures convert the images we see into nerve impulses?

    _____

13. Which structures allow us to see in color?

    _____

14. What is another term for the second cranial nerve?

    _____

15. Which term describes the area on the retina that produces the sharpest vision?

    _____

(Continued)

16. Which structure produces and excretes tears?

_____

17. When someone is crying, why might he or she experience a salty taste?

_____

18. What is the purpose of cerumen?

_____

Label the different parts of the ear in the following image.

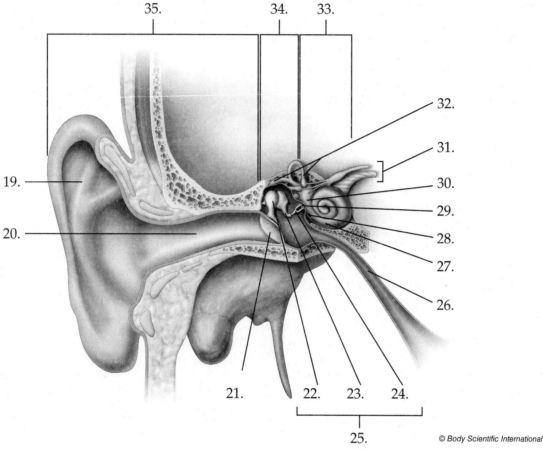

© Body Scientific International

19. _____   28. _____

20. _____   29. _____

21. _____   30. _____

22. _____   31. _____

23. _____   32. _____

24. _____   33. _____

25. _____   34. _____

26. _____   35. _____

27. _____

Understanding Terms Related to Diseases and Conditions

Match each of the following terms, which are related to conditions of the eye, to the correct meaning. You will not use all of the meanings.

_____ 1. exotropia

_____ 2. presbyopia

_____ 3. hyperopia

_____ 4. retinal detachment

_____ 5. hordeolum

_____ 6. cataract

_____ 7. vitreous floaters

_____ 8. glaucoma

_____ 9. dacryocystitis

_____ 10. entropion

_____ 11. myopia

_____ 12. astigmatism

_____ 13. esotropia

_____ 14. diabetic retinopathy

_____ 15. nystagmus

A. condition in which the eyelid turns inward

B. misalignment of the eyes in which one or both eyes turn inward

C. blockage, inflammation, and infection of the nasolacrimal duct and lacrimal sac

D. abnormal curvature of the cornea

E. repetitive, usually involuntary eye movement

F. condition caused by an increase in the pressure within the eyeball

G. condition caused by a shortened eyeball shape

H. clouding of the lens

I. condition in which one or both eyes turn outward

J. separation of the retina from its blood supply

K. deterioration of the macula as a result of the aging process

L. inflammation of an eyelid gland

M. damage to the retina due to diabetes mellitus

N. condition in which the eyeball is more elongated in shape than normal

O. farsightedness as a result of the aging process

P. the presence of specks or lines in the field of vision

Identify the term that corresponds to each disease or condition described below.

16. a fungal infection of the ear: _____

17. a ringing or buzzing sensation in the ears: _____

18. an impaired sense of taste: _____

19. a noncancerous tumor of the auditory nerve: _____

20. a disorder of the inner ear that results in vertigo: _____

21. a disease of the nerves: _____

22. hearing loss resulting from inadequate sound-wave conduction from the outer ear to bones of the middle ear: _____

23. a condition characterized by a weakened sense of smell: _____

(Continued)

24. a condition, seen commonly in children, in which the middle ear becomes inflamed:

_____

25. the condition in which the bones of the middle ear become hardened: _____

Match each of the following medical terms with the correct synonym. You will not use all of the synonyms.

_____ 26. anosmia

_____ 27. otomycosis

_____ 28. myopia

_____ 29. amblyopia

_____ 30. otalgia

_____ 31. cerumen

_____ 32. hyperopia

_____ 33. strabismus

_____ 34. ophthalmodynia

_____ 35. diplopia

A. double vision

B. earache

C. farsightedness

D. swimmer's ear

E. eye pain

F. earwax

G. crossed eyes

H. lazy eye

I. anosphrasia

J. normal vision

K. nearsightedness

L. saggy eyelid

Analyzing Diagnostic- and Treatment-Related Terms

Break down each of the following medical terms by rewriting the term, and then placing a slash between each word part (prefix, root word, combining vowel, and suffix if used). Then define each term.

1. audiometry

   Breakdown: _____

   Define: _____

2. graphesthesia

   Breakdown: _____

   Define: _____

3. photocoagulation

   Breakdown: _____

   Define: _____

4. myringotomy

   Breakdown: _____

   Define: _____

Read the following scenarios and answer the question in each one.

5. Jason has applied for a job with the police department. He must pass a physical exam before he can start work. One part of the exam is a test that assesses his visual clarity using a Snellen chart. What is the name of this test?

   _____

   _____

6. Another part of Jason's testing includes a series of neurological exams in which five kinds of responses are evaluated to identify problems with the CNS or PNS. What is the name of these tests?

   _____

   _____

7. Peter Turner is an audiologist whose assignment is to evaluate workers at an offshore oil rig for hearing problems. He knows that he will need a specific instrument to inspect the workers' external auditory canals and tympanic membranes. Which instrument is this, and for which test is it used?

   _____

   _____

(Continued)

8. Peter will also assess each worker's ability to detect sounds of different pitches. What equipment does he need for this test?

_____

_____

9. Peter is also expecting to perform a test that will assess the reactivity of the tympanic membrane to pressure changes. What is the name of this test, and which instrument does it require?

_____

_____

Laura is an RN in a busy HEENT specialist office. She is reviewing the patient roster for the day so that she can prepare exam rooms for the two doctors with whom she works.

10. The first patient of the day is a 3 y/o with recurrent otitis media, otalgia, and hypertrophy of the tonsils and adenoids. Laura knows the doctor will need to perform a visual examination of the patient's ears. What piece of equipment does Laura need to have available in this patient's exam room?

_____

_____

11. When Laura reviewed the chart for the 3 y/o patient, she noticed that the child has been taking medication to prevent a bacterial infection of the middle ear. What is this medication's classification?

_____

_____

12. When the doctor evaluates this patient, she decides that surgery is necessary to treat the condition. The doctor recommends a tonsillectomy and an adenoidectomy. She also recommends a procedure in which a surgical incision is made into the eardrum and a pressure-equalizing tube is placed in the tympanic membrane. What is the name of this procedure?

_____

_____

13. The next patient is a 6 y/o boy who suffered from sensorineural hearing loss at birth. He had surgery three weeks ago to have an electronic device that will restore his hearing surgically implanted in the inner ear. What is the name of this procedure?

_____

_____

(Continued)

14. Dr. Westmoreland, OD is starting a new practice in her hometown. What kind of specialist is Dr. Westmoreland?

_____

_____

15. While Dr. Westmoreland is unpacking her new equipment, she examines plates that will be used to test her patients for color blindness. In which test will these plates be used?

_____

_____

16. Dr. Westmoreland opens another box and finds the equipment she will use to examine the interior of her patients' eyes. What is the name of this test?

_____

_____

17. Next, she finds the equipment that is used to examine the front chamber of the eye with microscopic magnification. What is the name of this test?

_____

_____

18. There is also a box filled with pamphlets that contain information about surgery that will restore vision in the case of cataracts. What is the name of this surgery?

_____

_____

19. Dr. Reyes is an ophthalmologist who specializes in emergency cases. He receives a call from the ER about the victim of a gunshot wound to the face. The left side of the victim's face was affected, and the eye is unable to be saved. Which surgery would Dr. Reyes perform to remove the affected eyeball?

_____

_____

20. Later that day, Dr. Reyes receives a call from the ER concerning a patient who was admitted with c/o flashing lights and a shadow that obstructed his vision. Dr. Reyes knows that these symptoms are caused by retinal detachment. This condition requires immediate treatment or it will result in blindness. Which surgery is used to treat this condition?

_____

_____

Preparing for Your Future in Healthcare

Use the information on pages 275–276 of your textbook to define the following word parts.

1. acoust/o: _____

2. audi/o: _____

3. blephar/o: _____

4. cochle/o: _____

5. opt/o: _____

6. phac/o: _____

7. presby/o: _____

8. -cusis: _____

9. -opia: _____

10. -otia: _____

Use a regular or medical dictionary, the glossary in the back of your textbook, and your own words to define the following terms.

11. cochlear implant: _____

12. hyperopia: _____

13. myopia: _____

14. phacoemulsification: _____

15. presbycusis: _____

16. presbyopia: _____

17. vestibulocochlear nerve: _____

Match the appropriate healthcare professional with each of the following descriptions or tasks. You will use each profession more than once.

_____ 18. requires a degree from a medical school

_____ 19. treats patients with eye-related conditions

_____ 20. can perform surgery

_____ 21. may test newborns' hearing

_____ 22. can dispense contact lenses

_____ 23. treats patients with hearing-related conditions

_____ 24. treats children

_____ 25. can dispense hearing aids

A. optometrist
B. ophthalmologist
C. audiologist

Name _____ Date _____

Chapter 10 Practice Test

Using the word parts on pages 275–276 of your textbook, identify the medical term that corresponds to each of the following definitions.

1. inflammation of the eyelid: _____

2. disease of the retina: _____

3. "fear of," or sensitivity to, light: _____

4. hardening of the eardrum: _____

Break down each medical term listed below by rewriting the term, and then placing a slash between each word part (prefix, root word, combining vowel, and suffix if used). Then define each term.

5. aphakia

   Breakdown: _____

   Define: _____

6. keratotomy

   Breakdown: _____

   Define: _____

7. oculomycosis

   Breakdown: _____

   Define: _____

8. dacryocystocele

   Breakdown: _____

   Define: _____

9. retinoplasty

   Breakdown: _____

   Define: _____

10. mydriasis

   Breakdown: _____

   Define: _____

(Continued)

Answer the following questions.

11. Which five structures are generally considered organs of the special senses?

_____

_____

12. Which four structures protect the eyeball?

_____

_____

13. What substance gives the eye its shape?

_____

14. Which structures allow for peripheral vision?

_____

15. At what age do a person's lacrimal glands start producing tears?

_____

16. Which glands produce earwax?

_____

17. What is the term for the hammer-shaped bone in the middle ear?

_____

18. Which term describes the cells in the nose that allow a person to smell?

_____

19. What is the medical term for chewing?

_____

20. Where are the sensory receptors for touch located?

_____

_____

Identify the term that corresponds to each disease, condition, test, or procedure described below.

21. During a routine eye exam, an OD discovers that his patient has abnormally high intraocular pressure that has caused damage to the retina. Which term describes this condition?

_____

22. The doctor examines another patient who has a defective curvature of the cornea. What is this condition called?

_____

(Continued)

Name _____   Date _____

23. The next patient the doctor examines has a swollen, red eyelid gland that is filled with pus. Which term describes this condition?

_____

24. The first afternoon patient is scheduled for an eye test that will measure the area within which objects are seen when the eyes are in a fixed position. What is the name of this test?

_____

25. An ophthalmologist examines a patient who has been having difficulty with her vision, especially at night. The doctor notices that the patient's left lens is clouded. What diagnosis would the doctor write in this patient's chart?

_____

26. A medical assistant escorts a patient into the exam room. This patient is walking unsteadily and has to put her hands on the wall to prevent herself from falling. She states that she feels like the room is spinning. What term does the MA write in the patient's chart to describe her complaint?

_____

27. When the doctor examines this patient, he determines that her condition is caused by a disorder of the inner ear. Which term will the doctor use to describe this patient's condition?

_____

28. The next patient that the MA puts in the room has nasal congestion and rhinorrhea. He complains of being unable to taste anything. What term would the MA use to describe this condition?

_____

29. This same patient also complains of ear pain. What is the medical term for this condition?

_____

30. An Air Force flight surgeon is performing neurological testing of the pilots on his base. One of the tests that he performs requires a pilot to close his or her eyes and identify an object that is placed in his or her hand. This test is repeated with a different object in the other hand. What is the name of this test?

_____

Chapter 11

The Endocrine System

Name _____ Date _____

Understanding Word Parts

Match each of the following word parts with the correct meaning. You will not use all of the meanings.

_____ 1. -edema

_____ 2. -megaly

_____ 3. -dipsia

_____ 4. -assay

_____ 5. hypo-

_____ 6. poly-

_____ 7. -tropin

_____ 8. -oid

_____ 9. -uria

_____ 10. hyper-

A. urination; condition of urine

B. below; below normal; deficient

C. hormone

D. resembling

E. many; much

F. swelling; fluid retention

G. above; above normal; excessive

H. to analyze

I. pertaining to

J. thirst

K. enlargement

_____ 11. mast/o

_____ 12. myx/o

_____ 13. crin/o

_____ 14. kal/i

_____ 15. calc/o

_____ 16. ket/o

_____ 17. gonad/o

_____ 18. radi/o

_____ 19. gynec/o

_____ 20. cortic/o

A. sex glands

B. nerve

C. female; woman

D. X-rays

E. cortex

F. secrete

G. breast

H. potassium

I. mucus

J. ketone

K. calcium

(Continued)

Name _____   Date _____

Use the following combining forms and suffixes listed on pages 307–308 of your textbook to build the medical term that corresponds to each of the following definitions.

21. Word part: glyc/o

    Definition: condition of sugar in the urine

    Term: _____

22. Word part: tox/i

    Definition: condition of poison in the blood

    Term: _____

23. Word part: thyroid/o

    Definition: inflammation of the thyroid gland

    Term: _____

24. Word part: -ic

    Definition: pertaining to the eye

    Term: _____

25. Word part: thyr/o

    Definition: enlargement of the thyroid gland

    Term: _____

Break down each of the following medical terms by rewriting the term, and then placing a slash between each word part (prefix, root word, combining vowel, and suffix if used). Then define each term.

26. polydipsia

    Breakdown: _____

    Define: _____

27. hypoinsulinemia

    Breakdown: _____

    Define: _____

28. gigantism

    Breakdown: _____

    Define: _____

29. adrenocorticotropin

    Breakdown: _____

    Define: _____

30. hyperglycemia

    Breakdown: _____

    Define: _____

Interpreting Medical Records

Read the following medical record. Define the abbreviations and terms called out in the record, and then answer the questions that follow.

A-1C Endocrine Clinic

Dr. B. Shaw, **ATT PHY**

Patient Name: John Davidson

Date of Birth: 12/4/1963

Medical Record No.: DJ543

Subjective Data: A 54 y/o male presents to a clinic with c/o fatigue, tingling, and numbness in the **distal** lower extremities; **polydipsia**; **polyuria**; and **polyphagia**. Pt states that these symptoms began about a year ago after he changed jobs. At his current job, he spends most of the day at a desk.

PE: well-developed male; wt: 230 lbs; **P**: 72 **bpm**; **BP**: 144/92; **FBS**: 145 **mg/dL**; **GTT** results: 210 mmol/L

Dx: **hyperglycemia**, **NIDDM**, **obesity**, borderline **HTN**

Tx: Start pt on Metformin 500 **mg b.i.d.**

Dispense home glucose monitor and check blood sugar levels **q.i.d.**, **a.c.**, and **h.s.**

Consult with **CDE** for diet counseling and disease management

Refer to **CFT** for exercise plan

Set up pt for **EKG** to R/O **CAD**

Pt to return to clinic every week to recheck BP and FBS

Follow up with Dr. Shaw in 3 months

---

1. ATT PHY: _____

2. distal: _____

3. polydipsia: _____

4. polyuria: _____

5. polyphagia: _____

6. P: _____

7. bpm: _____

8. BP: _____

9. FBS: _____

10. mg/dl: _____

11. GTT: _____

12. Dx: _____

13. hyperglycemia: _____

(Continued)

14. NIDDM: _____

15. obesity: _____

16. HTN: _____

17. tx: _____

18. mg: _____

19. b.i.d.: _____

20. q.i.d.: _____

21. a.c.: _____

22. h.s.: _____

23. consult: _____

24. CDE: _____

25. CFT: _____

26. EKG: _____

27. CAD: _____

28. When is Mr. Davidson supposed to check his blood sugar levels at home?

_____

_____

29. Which complaint indicates that Mr. Davidson may be developing complications related to his diagnosis?

_____

_____

30. Which medical term describes the complaint referenced in the previous question?

_____

_____

Comprehending Anatomy and Physiology Terminology

Use a regular or medical dictionary, the glossary in the back of your textbook, and your own words to define the following terms.

1. circadian rhythm: _____

2. cortex: _____

3. gland: _____

4. medulla: _____

5. tropins: _____

Answer the following questions.

6. List the primary organs and glands of the endocrine system.

_____

7. Which gland controls all the other endocrine glands?

_____

8. Which gland is important in regulating the body's "sleep-and-waking" cycle?

_____

9. Which two glands are located in the throat?

_____

10. Which two hormones, secreted by the thyroid and the parathyroid glands, counteract each other?

_____

11. Which cells secrete the hormone that helps lower blood sugar?

_____

12. Which cells secrete the hormone that helps raise blood sugar?

_____

13. What is the medical term for sex cells?

_____

14. Which term describes the female gonads?

_____

15. What causes a male's voice to develop a deeper sound?

_____

(Continued)

Match each of the following hormones with the correct function. You will not use all of the functions.

_____ 16. ACTH

_____ 17. ADH

_____ 18. aldosterone

_____ 19. calcitonin

_____ 20. cortisol

_____ 21. epinephrine

_____ 22. FSH

_____ 23. GH

_____ 24. insulin

_____ 25. LH

_____ 26. MSH

_____ 27. oxytocin

_____ 28. progesterone

_____ 29. TSH

_____ 30. T_3

A. helps regulate puberty

B. helps maintain pregnancy

C. stimulates the deposit of calcium into the bones and lowers blood calcium levels

D. stimulates uterine contractions during childbirth and the release of milk in females who are breastfeeding

E. stimulates the production of cortisol

F. triggers the body's fight-or-flight response

G. regulates blood pressure, electrolyte levels, and fluid volume

H. controls metabolism and body temperature

I. stimulates ovulation and controls menstruation

J. stimulates the kidneys to retain water and constricts blood vessels

K. regulates the absorption of glucose into blood cells

L. regulates the release of TSH

M. stimulates the thyroid gland and helps regulate thyroid function

N. stimulates the production of skin pigment

O. regulates blood glucose levels and helps metabolize carbohydrates, proteins, and fats

P. stimulates body growth and development

Name _____ Date _____

Understanding Terms Related to Diseases and Conditions

Break down each of the following medical terms by rewriting the term, and then placing a slash between each word part (prefix, root word, combining vowel, and suffix if used). Then define each term.

1. acidosis

   Breakdown: _____

   Define: _____

   _____

   _____

2. adenocarcinoma

   Breakdown: _____

   Define: _____

   _____

   _____

3. gynecomastia

   Breakdown: _____

   Define: _____

   _____

   _____

4. hyperparathyroidism

   Breakdown: _____

   Define: _____

   _____

   _____

5. hyponatremia

   Breakdown: _____

   Define: _____

   _____

   _____

(Continued)

Name _____   Date _____

Read the following scenarios and answer the question in each one.

Imagine that you are job shadowing Ruth, an RN who is the head office nurse for Dr. White, an endocrinologist. Ruth is reviewing the patient roster for the day.

6. The first patient of the morning is Joe. According to the new patient information sheet, Joe is a former body builder. While reviewing the referral from Joe's primary care physician, you notice she has requested an evaluation by Dr. White because Joe has recently gained a lot of weight. Joe's listed weight is 20% more than the average for his age, gender, build, and height. Which term describes this condition?

_____

7. On the lab reports provided by his PCP, Joe's cortisol levels are well above what is considered normal for him. Ruth calls Joe back into the room so that she can take his vital signs. Ruth weighs Joe and you notice that his ankles and feet are swollen. Which medical term describes this condition?

_____

8. You also notice that Joe has several bruises on his legs and arms. Ruth takes Joe's blood pressure and records the result in his chart as 150/100. You remember from class that anything above 140/90 is considered higher than normal. What term would you expect Ruth to use to describe Joe's blood pressure reading?

_____

9. Dr. White comes into the room to examine Joe. During the interview, Joe tells Dr. White that he used anabolic steroids for several years. He states that he has not used any steroids in over six months. Joe complains of feeling weak and not having the energy he had when using steroids. What do you think Dr. White's diagnosis for Joe will be?

_____

10. The next appointment is an urgent evaluation for Andrea, a 35-year-old female who was admitted to the ER last night with extreme anxiety and muscle spasms. Lab work performed in the ER shows that Andrea's blood calcium levels are well below normal. Which term describes the muscle condition Andrea was experiencing while in the ER?

_____

11. Ruth escorts Andrea into an exam room. During the interview, Andrea tells Ruth that she suffered a fracture of her distal fibula three months ago. Ruth reviews the X-ray and notices that the bone seems to have healed without any complications. However, Andrea's orthopedic specialist ordered a bone density test and the results showed significant bone loss, especially for Andrea's age. Dr. White reviews the lab work from the ER and notices that Andrea's PTH level is elevated. What do you think is Andrea's diagnosis?

_____

(Continued)

12. Jean is a 54-year-old female with complaints of unexpected weight loss and abnormal anxiety. She was evaluated by her PCP, who referred her to Dr. White. While Ruth is weighing the patient, you notice that Jean's face looks peculiar. You look closer and notice that Jean's eyes are bulging slightly and appear larger than you would expect. Which term describes this condition?

_____

13. Dr. White palpates Jean's neck and tells Ruth to document hypertrophy of the thyroid gland. What does this mean?

_____

_____

14. While reviewing the lab reports on Jean's chart, you notice that her T_3 and T_4 levels are elevated. Which term describes this condition?

_____

15. Dr. White explains to Jean that she has an autoimmune condition that has caused her thyroid gland to become overactive. Which medical term describes this diagnosis?

_____

16. Andy is a 19 y/o male who has had DM since childhood. Now, as a college student, he is not managing his condition as well as he did when he was at home. Andy requires insulin injections q.i.d. and sometimes he "forgets" to check his blood sugar. Which term describes Andy's condition?

_____

17. Dr. White tells Andy that he is going to have to treat his hyperglycemia or he will have complications. What does the term *hyperglycemia* mean?

_____

_____

_____

18. You remember learning about a condition in which the retina of the eye can be damaged as a complication of DM. Which term describes this condition?

_____

19. Dr. White explains to Andy that he may also start experiencing pain and weakness, especially in his hands and feet. Which term describes this condition?

_____

20. Andy tells Dr. White that he recently spent three days in the hospital. Andy said the doctor told him that he had an acute episode of diabetic ketoacidosis. Andy asked Dr. White to explain this condition to him. What would you expect Dr. White to tell Andy?

_____

_____

Analyzing Diagnostic- and Treatment-Related Terms

Match each of the following terms with the correct meaning. You will not use all of the meanings.

_____ 1. catecholamines test

_____ 2. FBS

_____ 3. quantitative HCG test

_____ 4. TSH test

_____ 5. thyroid ultrasound

_____ 6. T$_3$RU test

_____ 7. qualitative HCG test

_____ 8. T$_4$ test

_____ 9. PBI test

_____ 10. T$_3$ test

_____ 11. GTT

_____ 12. thyroid scan

A. test that measures the amounts of thyroxine in the blood by testing for levels of triiodothyronine

B. test that measures the glucose levels in a patient's blood

C. test in which a camera is used to record the accumulation of a radioactive chemical as it moves into the thyroid

D. test that measures the amount of glucose in the blood after a patient has eaten a large meal

E. test that requires a patient to collect his or her urine for 24 hours

F. test that determines the amount of protein-bound iodine in the blood

G. test in which a sugar solution is administered to a patient before blood is drawn at timed intervals

H. test considered to be the most accurate for measuring thyroid activity

I. test that measures the amount of triiodothyronine in the blood

J. test that measures the amount of human chorionic gonadotropin in the blood

K. test that uses sound waves to produce a visual image of the endocrine gland in the throat

L. test that measures the amount of thyroxine in the blood

M. test that determines whether a woman is pregnant

Identify the term that corresponds to each procedure or treatment described below.

13. What might be a treatment option for a 10-year-old male with a diagnosis of dwarfism?

_____

_____

14. What is a possible treatment option for a 53-year-old female with Graves' disease and exophthalmos?

_____

_____

15. Which drug treatment should be used for a 6-year-old female with a diagnosis of IDDM?

_____

_____

Preparing for Your Future in Healthcare

Define each of the following abbreviations.

1. CDE: _____

2. DI: _____

3. FBS: _____

4. IDDM: _____

5. NIDDM: _____

6. SIADH: _____

Use a regular or medical dictionary, the glossary in the back of your textbook, and your own words to define the following terms.

7. hormones: _____

8. infertility: _____

9. menopause: _____

10. phlebotomy: _____

Match the appropriate healthcare professional with each of the following descriptions or tasks. You will use each profession more than once.

A. nutritionist   B. endocrinologist   C. certified diabetes educator   D. phlebotomist

_____ 11. assists people with diet planning

_____ 12. requires a degree from a medical school

_____ 13. may work in a school

_____ 14. requires some college coursework

_____ 15. may work in a blood bank

_____ 16. may educate people with IDDM on how to administer their medications

_____ 17. generally receives on-the-job training during coursework

_____ 18. may treat women experiencing infertility

_____ 19. will prepare blood to be sent to the laboratory

_____ 20. requires a state license

Name _____ Date _____

Chapter 11 Practice Test

Identify the term that corresponds to each disease or condition described below.

1. condition of deficient glucose in the blood: _____

2. condition of excessive potassium in the blood: _____

3. the surgical removal of a breast: _____

4. condition of excessive urination: _____

Break down each medical term listed below by rewriting the term, and then placing a slash between each word part (prefix, root word, combining vowel, and suffix if used). Then define each term.

5. retinoblastoma

    Breakdown: _____

    Define: _____

6. panhypopituitarism

    Breakdown: _____

    Define: _____

7. thyrotoxicosis

    Breakdown: _____

    Define: _____

Match each of the following terms with the correct meaning. You will not use all of the meanings.

_____ 8. adenocarcinoma

_____ 9. type 2 diabetes

_____ 10. pheochromocytoma

_____ 11. diabetic ketoacidosis

_____ 12. Addison's disease

_____ 13. acidosis

_____ 14. diabetes insipidus

_____ 15. dwarfism

_____ 16. gynecomastia

A. condition of being smaller or shorter than normal

B. disease caused by insufficient secretion of cortisol and sometimes aldosterone

C. tumor of the adrenal gland that secretes excess epinephrine and norepinephrine

D. disease caused by inadequate secretion of ADH by the posterior pituitary gland

E. a malignant tumor of any gland or mucus-secreting organ

F. tumor of the beta cells of the islets of Langerhans, which causes an increase in the secretion of insulin

G. condition in which the body produces acidic ketone bodies as a result of high blood glucose levels

H. general term that describes any condition in which the body experiences an increase in the acidity of the blood, body fluids, or tissues

I. disease in which insulin production is normal, but the body cannot use the insulin efficiently

J. condition in which a male develops abnormally large mammary glands

(Continued)

Define each of the following abbreviations for hormones, and then indicate which gland in the endocrine system secretes the hormone.

17. ACTH

   Meaning: _____

   Gland: _____

18. ADH

   Meaning: _____

   Gland: _____

19. CRH

   Meaning: _____

   Gland: _____

20. FSH

   Meaning: _____

   Gland: _____

21. GH

   Meaning: _____

   Gland: _____

22. GHIH

   Meaning: _____

   Gland: _____

23. GHRH

   Meaning: _____

   Gland: _____

24. GnRH

   Meaning: _____

   Gland: _____

25. MSH

   Meaning: _____

   Gland: _____

(Continued)

26. PTH

    Meaning: _____

    Gland: _____

27. T_3

    Meaning: _____

    Gland: _____

28. T_4

    Meaning: _____

    Gland: _____

29. TRH

    Meaning: _____

    Gland: _____

30. TSH

    Meaning: _____

    Gland: _____

Chapter 12

The Urinary System

Name _____ Date _____

Understanding Word Parts

Match each of the following word parts with the correct meaning. You will not use all of the meanings.

_____ 1. inter-

_____ 2. -poietin

_____ 3. -cele

_____ 4. -iasis

_____ 5. -sclerosis

_____ 6. -lysis

_____ 7. -uria

_____ 8. -tripsy

_____ 9. an-

_____ 10. -pexy

A. hernia; swelling; protrusion

B. urination; condition of urine

C. breakdown; separation; loosening

D. substance that forms

E. crushing

F. between

G. hardening; thickening

H. surgical fixation

I. structure; tissue; thing

J. not; without

K. abnormal condition

_____ 11. olig/o

_____ 12. cali/o

_____ 13. pyel/o

_____ 14. azot/o

_____ 15. meat/o

_____ 16. nephr/o

_____ 17. cyst/o

_____ 18. noct/o

_____ 19. bacteri/o

_____ 20. vesic/o

A. peritoneum

B. cyst; fluid sac; bladder

C. meatus

D. nitrogen

E. bacteria

F. night

G. kidney

H. urinary bladder

I. scanty

J. calyx

K. renal pelvis

(Continued)

Name _____ Date _____

Use the following combining forms and suffixes listed on pages 335–336 of your textbook to build the medical term that corresponds to each of the following definitions.

21. Word part: -ar

    Definition: pertaining to the glomerulus

    Term: _____

22. Word part: nephr/o

    Definition: hardening or thickening of the kidney

    Term: _____

23. Word part: cyst/o

    Definition: inflammation of the bladder

    Term: _____

Break down each of the following medical terms by rewriting the term, and then placing a slash between each word part (prefix, root word, combining vowel, and suffix if used). Then define each term.

24. cystoscopy

    Breakdown: _____

    Define: _____

25. dialysis

    Breakdown: _____

    Define: _____

26. nephrectomy

    Breakdown: _____

    Define: _____

27. genitourinary

    Breakdown: _____

    Define: _____

28. ureterostenosis

    Breakdown: _____

    Define: _____

29. cystolithotomy

    Breakdown: _____

    Define: _____

(Continued)

30. nephropexy

   Breakdown: _____

   Define: _____

31. hydronephrosis

   Breakdown: _____

   Define: _____

32. anuria

   Breakdown: _____

   Define: _____

33. hematuria

   Breakdown: _____

   Define: _____

34. urethrospasm

   Breakdown: _____

   Define: _____

35. retroperitoneal

   Breakdown: _____

   Define: _____

Interpreting Medical Records

Read the following medical record. Define the abbreviations and medical terms called out in the record, and then answer the questions that follow.

<u>Kidney Wellness Center</u>

<u>Dr. Amy Murphy</u>

Patient Name: Mary Sanders

Date of Birth: 3-12-1985

Medical Record No.: 56347

Date of Exam: 5-3-2017

Subjective Data: **Pt** is a 32 **y/o** female who had a normal vaginal delivery of her third child nine months ago. There were no complications with the pregnancy, labor, or delivery. She has **c/o incontinence** since the birth. Pt has tried exercise but symptoms have not improved. She must wear a pad at all times. She has stopped running because she is worried about having an accident before she can reach a bathroom. Because she has not been able to exercise as much as she did before having her last child, she has gained about 20 lbs. Pt was evaluated by **OB/GYN** and her uterus was found to be **WNL**. Pt was referred to urology for evaluation and recommendation of **tx** options. Pt is a **NS**.

Objective Data: **wt**: 160 lbs; **ht**: 65″; **P**: 76; **R**: 14; **T**: 97.6°; **BP**: 120/64

HEENT: WNL

CV Hx: not significant

GU *Hx*: Three pregnancies, three live births, all delivered vaginally without complications. No recent history of **UTI** or **nephrolithiasis**. Pt reports that she uses about four pads a day, depending on her activity level. Pt states that leakage increases with sneezing or laughing. Pt denies **dysuria**, **hematuria**, and **polyuria**. No changes in medication noted. Pt has no history of abdominal surgery.

PE: **Cystocele** noted with vaginal examination.

Assessment: Grade 1 cystocele. **Internal urethral sphincter** deficiency.

Recommendation: Collect urine via straight in-and-out **CATH** for **UA**.

Schedule Pt for **VCUG**.

Refer Pt to **PT** for recommendation and teaching exercises to strength pelvic floor muscles.

---

1. Pt: _____

2. y/o: _____

3. c/o: _____

4. incontinence: _____

    _____

    _____

5. OB/GYN: _____

(Continued)

Name _____   Date _____

6. WNL: _____

7. tx: _____

8. NS: _____

9. wt: _____

10. ht: _____

11. P: _____

12. R: _____

13. T: _____

14. BP: _____

15. HEENT: _____

16. CV: _____

17. Hx: _____

18. GU: _____

19. UTI: _____

20. nephrolithiasis: _____

_____

_____

21. dysuria: _____

_____

_____

22. hematuria: _____

_____

_____

23. polyuria: _____

_____

_____

24. PE: _____

25. cystocele: _____

_____

_____

(Continued)

26. internal urethral sphincter: _____

_____

_____

27. CATH: _____

28. UA: _____

29. VCUG: _____

30. PT: _____

31. Why do you think this patient is experiencing incontinence?

_____

_____

_____

_____

Imagine that you work as a student intern in the laboratory at UMC hospital. You have just received the samples for several doctor's offices. Which test is indicated by each of the following abbreviations?

32. BUN: _____

33. CBC: _____

34. Hct: _____

35. Hgb: _____

36. GFR: _____

37. pH: _____

38. FBS: _____

39. PKU: _____

40. sp gr: _____

Comprehending Anatomy and Physiology Terminology

Use a regular or medical dictionary, the glossary in the back of your textbook, and your own words to define the following terms.

1. filtration: _____

_____

2. excretion: _____

_____

3. ions: _____

_____

4. homeostasis: _____

_____

5. urinary tract: _____

_____

6. electrolytes: _____

_____

7. urination: _____

_____

8. nephron: _____

_____

9. filtrate: _____

_____

10. urea: _____

_____

Using the information on pages 335–336, define the following word parts.

11. cyst/o: _____

12. glomerul/o: _____

13. peritone/o: _____

14. pyel/o: _____

15. ureter/o: _____

16. retro-: _____

(Continued)

Name _____ Date _____

Answer the following questions.

17. What are the four main functions of the urinary system?

_____

_____

18. Which hormone produced by the kidneys stimulates hematopoiesis?

_____

19. List the three ways in which the kidneys help the body maintain homeostasis.

_____

_____

20. Which term describes the area behind the membranous lining of the abdominopelvic cavity?

_____

21. Which three terms are used to describe the discharge of urine from the bladder?

_____

Label the parts of the kidney in the following image.

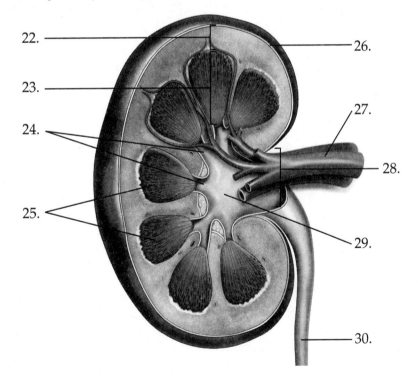

© *Body Scientific International*

22. _____   27. _____

23. _____   28. _____

24. _____   29. _____

25. _____   30. _____

26. _____

Understanding Terms Related to Diseases and Conditions

Match each of the following medical terms with the correct meaning. You will not use all of the meanings.

_____ 1. urinary incontinence

_____ 2. polyuria

_____ 3. hematuria

_____ 4. oliguria

_____ 5. urinary retention

_____ 6. diuresis

_____ 7. glycosuria

_____ 8. anuria

_____ 9. enuresis

_____ 10. urinary urgency

_____ 11. dysuria

_____ 12. nocturnal enuresis

A. the presence of sugars in the urine

B. the presence of blood in the urine

C. difficult or painful urination

D. loss of voluntary control over the discharge of urine from the bladder

E. an inability to completely empty the bladder

F. the presence of stones in the urine

G. condition of excessive urine production

H. absence of urine production

I. bed wetting

J. involuntary discharge of urine

K. condition in which a small amount of urine is produced

L. the sudden, urgent need to urinate

M. abnormal increase in the production of urine

Identify the term that corresponds to each disease or condition described below.

13. inflammation of the lining of the renal pelvis and the kidney: _____

14. inflammation of the bladder: _____

15. inflammation of the glomeruli in the kidney: _____

16. chronic inflammation of the bladder wall: _____

17. condition of stones in the kidney: _____

18. condition of stones in the bladder: _____

19. condition in which the bladder protrudes through a weakened place in the vaginal wall:

_____

20. condition in which an abnormal opening forms between the bladder and vagina: _____

21. cancerous tumor of the kidney in a 65 y/o male: _____

22. cancerous tumor of the kidney in a 5 y/o male: _____

23. condition of the kidney in which damage or disease causes impaired filtration: _____

24. condition in which the arteriole walls of the kidneys become narrowed and thickened:

_____

25. condition characterized by the development of fluid-filled sacs within the kidney, leading to

nephromegaly: _____

Name _____   Date _____

Analyzing Diagnostic- and Treatment-Related Terms

Imagine that you are a certified medical assistant (CMA) working in a busy specialists' office. The providers in this office include Dr. Cindy Pate, a urologist; Dr. Sam Greene, a nephrologist; and Dr. Tamera Lyons, an endocrinologist. One of your most common tasks is to perform an in-office UA on almost every patient. It is important for you to know the normal results for a UA. Identify what you would expect to be normal for each of the following observations that you make when performing this test.

1. color: _____

   _____

2. pH: _____

   _____

3. protein: _____

   _____

4. glucose: _____

   _____

5. ketones: _____

   _____

6. occult hematuria: _____

   _____

7. leukocytes: _____

   _____

8. nitrates: _____

   _____

9. bilirubin: _____

   _____

Read the following scenarios and answer the questions.

10. In addition to the UA, you routinely perform a test that requires you to spin a urine sample in a special machine to separate the urine's solids from its liquid. What is the name of the machine that you would use for this test?

    _____

11. You also educate your patients about a test that requires them to collect their urine for a 24-hour period and take it to the lab, where it will be tested along with a sample of the patient's blood to determine how well the glomeruli in the kidneys are functioning. What is the name of this test?

    _____

(Continued)

12. You routinely draw blood and send it to the lab to measure the amount of waste products in the blood. What is the name of this test?

_____

13. You review the patient list for the day to make sure you have all of the test results ready for the doctors to review before they see their patients. The first chart you check for Dr. Pate is a patient who had an X-ray test in which the kidneys, ureters, and bladder were viewed using a contrast agent. What is the name of this test?

_____

14. Dr. Greene has a patient named Bob Gomez who has recently had a shunt placed in his left forearm so that he can undergo treatments that will filter his blood through a machine and return cleansed blood to his system. What is the name for this treatment?

_____

15. Mr. Gomez had a test performed to evaluate the blood vessels of his kidney. This test uses a contrast medium and a camera that records the flow of blood. What is the name of this test?

_____

16. Mr. Gomez had this test performed because he will soon be added to a list of people waiting to receive a donor kidney. What procedure will Mr. Gomez undergo if he receives a donor kidney?

_____

17. Dr. Lyons is seeing a patient named Mrs. Wilma Robinson. Mrs. Robinson has lived with IDDM for 25 years. She has also been dealing with a chronic UTI for the past six months. She has been taking medication to treat this condition, but the infection keeps coming back. Which classification of medication should she be taking to treat this infection?

_____

18. Dr. Lyons has consulted with Dr. Pate concerning Mrs. Robinson. They decided that Dr. Pate would perform a visual examination of the urinary bladder to identify any abnormalities. What is the name of this test?

_____

19. While reviewing Mrs. Robinson's chart, you discover that she received treatment for a bladder stone three years ago. This treatment used high-energy shockwaves to break up the stone. What is the name of this treatment?

_____

20. After this treatment, Mrs. Robinson went home with a flexible tube placed in her bladder. The tube exited through her urethra so that her bladder would not fill up with urine. What is the name of this procedure?

_____

(Continued)

21. Jerry McDaniel is a patient of Dr. Pate's who recently had a kidney removed due to polycystic kidney disease. What is the name of this surgery?

_____

22. Jerry has developed some lower extremity edema. To treat this problem, Dr. Pate is going to put Jerry on a trial of a medication that will increase his urine output. What is the classification of this medication?

_____

23. Dr. Pate wants to schedule Jerry for a test that will determine how his remaining kidney is functioning. This test is an X-ray visualization of the renal pelvis, ureters, and bladder using a contrast medium. What is the name of this test?

_____

24. Dr. Greene's next patient is Tyler, a six-year-old male who was diagnosed with a Wilms tumor. This diagnosis came after a procedure in which a small amount of the tumor's tissue was removed from the kidney using a hollow needle to be evaluated by a pathologist. What is the name of this procedure?

_____

25. Dr. Greene wants Tyler to undergo a radiographic test in which images of the kidney and abdominal area are taken from multiple angles using a contrast medium and analyzed by a computer. What is the name of this procedure?

_____

Preparing for Your Future in Healthcare

Using the information on pages 335–336, define the following word parts.

1. iatr/o: _____

2. -ic: _____

3. -logist: _____

4. nephr/o: _____

5. onc/o: _____

6. ur/o: _____

Use a regular or medical dictionary, the glossary in the back of your textbook, and your own words to define the following terms.

7. dialysis: _____

8. nephrologist: _____

9. oncologist: _____

10. urologist: _____

Match the appropriate healthcare professional with each of the following descriptions. You will use each profession more than once.

    A. dialysis technician   B. urologist   C. case management nurse

_____ 11. I must receive orders from a doctor or nurse before I can begin my treatments.

_____ 12. I graduated from nursing school.

_____ 13. I have my own private practice.

_____ 14. I operate equipment designed to eliminate toxins from the blood of patients whose kidneys are not functioning properly.

_____ 15. I may visit a patient in his or her home.

_____ 16. I must pass a test given by BONENT before I can work.

_____ 17. I graduated from medical school.

_____ 18. I can only work in a hospital or outpatient clinic setting.

_____ 19. I coordinate a patient's care with other members of the healthcare team.

_____ 20. I can treat bladder cancer.

_____ 21. I graduated from a technical school.

_____ 22. I can receive a certification from ACMA.

_____ 23. I can perform surgery for male sterilization.

_____ 24. I can receive certification from NNCO.

_____ 25. It is important that I understand the cost of a patient's healthcare needs.

Chapter 12 Practice Test

Using the word parts on pages 335–336 of your textbook, identify the medical term that corresponds to each of the following definitions.

1. condition of scanty urination: _____

2. condition of much urination: _____

3. condition of pus in the urine: _____

4. surgical repair of the ureter: _____

5. inflammation of the peritoneum: _____

Break down each medical term listed below by rewriting the term, and then placing a slash between each word part (prefix, root word, combining vowel, and suffix if used). Then define each term.

6. nephromegaly

   Breakdown: _____

   Define: _____

7. ureterolithiasis

   Breakdown: _____

   Define: _____

8. cystorrhaphy

   Breakdown: _____

   Define: _____

9. vesicotomy

   Breakdown: _____

   Define: _____

10. azotemia

    Breakdown: _____

    Define: _____

Answer the following questions.

11. Define the term *filtration*.

    _____

    _____

    _____

(Continued)

12. What is the function of calcitriol, a hormone produced by the kidneys?

_____

_____

13. List the three regions of the kidney.

_____

14. Where are the functional units of the kidney located?

_____

15. In which part of the nephron does reabsorption take place?

_____

16. What are the five major components of urine?

_____

_____

17. Which term describes the depression in a kidney that serves as a passageway for blood vessels, lymphatic vessels, and nerves?

_____

18. Approximately how much volume can the urinary bladder hold before the brain is notified that it is time to be emptied?

_____

19. How long is the female urethra?

_____

Identify the term that corresponds to each disease or condition described below.

20. scanty urination:

_____

21. no urine production:

_____

22. presence of blood in the urine:

_____

23. difficult or painful urination:

_____

24. involuntary discharge of urine at night:

_____

(Continued)

Identify the correct diagnosis for each patient described below.

25. 35 y/o male with symptoms of hyperglycemia, polydipsia, polyuria, and deficiency of insulin in the blood:

_____

26. 45 y/o female with multiple cysts in the kidney accompanied by nephromegaly:

_____

27. 28 y/o male with severe lower back pain and positive X-ray for renal calculi:

_____

Identify the correct test or treatment described in each situation below.

28. treatment in which high-energy shock waves are used to attempt to break up renal calculi:

_____

29. an examination of the urine to test for abnormal elements:

_____

30. removal of the kidney:

_____

Chapter 13

The Male Reproductive System

Name _____ Date _____

Understanding Word Parts

Match each of the following word parts with the correct meaning. You will not use all of the meanings.

_____ 1. -pexy

_____ 2. -megaly

_____ 3. -trophy

_____ 4. -genesis

_____ 5. -rrhea

_____ 6. hypo-

_____ 7. trans-

_____ 8. -lytic

_____ 9. peri-

_____ 10. -stomy

A. below; below normal; deficient

B. formation

C. across

D. pertaining to breakdown or destruction

E. flow; excessive discharge

F. condition of growth or development

G. around; surrounding

H. surgical opening

I. structure; tissue; thing

J. enlargement

K. surgical fixation

_____ 11. vas/o

_____ 12. gyn/o

_____ 13. mast/o

_____ 14. andr/o

_____ 15. zo/o

_____ 16. crypt/o

_____ 17. onc/o

_____ 18. balan/o

_____ 19. vener/o

_____ 20. orchi/o

A. female; woman

B. cold

C. male

D. vessel; duct

E. hidden

F. testis

G. glans penis

H. animal; life

I. tumor

J. sexual contact

K. breast

(Continued)

Name _____ Date _____

Use the following combining forms listed on pages 363–364 of your textbook to build the medical term that corresponds to each of the following definitions.

21. Word part: spermat/o

    Definition: formation of sperm

    Term: _____

22. Word part: orchi/o

    Definition: surgical fixation of a testicle

    Term: _____

23. Word part: sperm/o

    Definition: pertaining to the destruction of sperm

    Term: _____

Break down each of the following medical terms by rewriting the term, and then placing a slash between each word part (prefix, root word, combining vowel, and suffix if used). Then define each term.

24. azoospermia

    Breakdown: _____

    Define: _____

25. anorchism

    Breakdown: _____

    Define: _____

26. transrectal

    Breakdown: _____

    Define: _____

27. prostatovesiculitis

    Breakdown: _____

    Define: _____

28. electrocautery

    Breakdown: _____

    Define: _____

29. andropathy

    Breakdown: _____

    Define: _____

30. balanoplasty

    Breakdown: _____

    Define: _____

Interpreting Medical Records

Read the following medical record. Define the abbreviations and terms called out in the record, and then answer the questions that follow.

Sunshine Valley Urology Clinic

Dr. Gary Thomas, MD

3100 N. Happy Trails Drive, Ste 250

Sunnyville, CO 12345

PMH: 52 y/o male with Hx of **NIDDM** for 15 years. Pt manages condition with oral medications. **FBS** ranges from 80 to 138 **mg/dl** for the past three months. Pt has not complained of changes in **VA** and states that he is evaluated annually by his **ophthalmologist**. Pt has started noticing numbness and tingling in his toes, especially when his blood sugar is greater than 120 mg/dl. Pt has recently experienced difficulty achieving and maintaining an erection during sexual activity. Pt was evaluated by PCP and **endocrinologist**, and then referred to the urology department for evaluation and Tx.

SH: Pt is a **NS** and denies frequent alcohol consumption, although he admits to having an occasional beer with his friends about once a month. Pt denies recreational drug use.

OH: Pt is a high school math teacher.

FH: Pt's father had a **Dx** of **DM** for 40 years and passed away at age 70 of a **MI**. Pt's mother has a Dx of **AD** and is living in a nursing home. Pt has two brothers who are living—one, age 56, has a Dx of **CAD** and **CHF**, and the other, age 58, suffers from **COPD**. Pt had a sister who passed away at age 35 of **SLE**.

Psychosocial: Pt has been married to same spouse for 24 years. They have spent the past 10 summers serving on various overseas church mission trips. Pt and his spouse have three adult children together. One child is in the military and is currently overseas. Their middle child is married and has two children. Their youngest child is in college. Pt admits that the burden of caring for his aging mother, having a child in college, and having another child overseas in the military has caused a mental and financial burden, but he states, "I think I am handling it well." Pt does admit that his inability to achieve an erection has caused him some anxiety, but he states that his spouse is very understanding.

PE: ht: 72 inches; wt: 191.2 pounds

HEENT: deferred

CV: P: 74 bpm; **BP**: 152/92; heart sounds: WNL

Dorsal pedal pulses slightly less predominant than radial and carotid pulses, bilaterally. Normal rate and rhythm of pulses.

GU: Circumcised penis noted without discharge or abnormalities. Scrotal sac appears WNL. **DRE** reveals a normally sized prostate gland. Pt denies **dysuria**, **nocturia**, or **hematuria**. Recent ultrasound of genitals reveals a mild decrease in blood flow to the penis.

Lab: **CBC** is WNL

Kidney and liver function is WNL

Testosterone, **LH**, **FSH**, prolactin, T_3, T_4, and **TSH** are all WNL

Cholesterol: 215 mg/dl

Impression: Dx of **ED** secondary to DM

Plan: Recommend a low fat/low cholesterol diet. Refer back to PCP for evaluation of **HTN**. Trial of sildenafil with 50 mg **p.o.** daily, to be taken about 30 minutes to 4 h prior to sexual activity. Pharmacist to educate pt on side effects and precautions involved with this medication. Pt should follow up in four months, or sooner if indicated.

(Continued)

Name _____   Date _____

1. PMH: _____   18. SLE: _____

2. NIDDM: _____   19. CV: _____

3. FBS: _____   20. BP: _____

4. mg/dl: _____   21. DRE: _____

5. VA: _____   22. dysuria: _____

6. ophthalmologist: _____   _____

_____   23. nocturia: _____

7. endocrinologist: _____   _____

_____   24. hematuria: _____

8. SH: _____   _____

9. NS: _____   25. CBC: _____

10. FH: _____   26. LH: _____

11. Dx: _____   27. FSH: _____

12. DM: _____   28. T_3: _____

13. MI: _____   29. T_4: _____

14. AD: _____   30. TSH: _____

15. CAD: _____   31. ED: _____

16. CHF: _____   32. HTN: _____

17. COPD: _____   33. p.o.: _____

34. Describe where you would find each of the following pulses.

dorsal pedal pulse: _____

radial pulse: _____

carotid pulse: _____

35. What did the urologist determine in his physical examination that caused him to refer this patient back to his PCP?

_____

Comprehending Anatomy and Physiology Terminology

Use a regular or medical dictionary, the glossary in the back of your textbook, and your own words to define the following terms.

1. sperm: _____

2. spermatogenesis: _____

3. semen: _____

4. puberty: _____

5. ejaculation: _____

Using the information on pages 363–364 of your textbook, define the following word parts.

6. balan/o: _____

7. orchi/o: _____

8. semin/o: _____

9. test/o: _____

10. vas/o: _____

Label the parts of the testis and epididymis in the following image.

11. _____

12. _____

13. _____

14. _____

15. _____

16. _____

17. _____

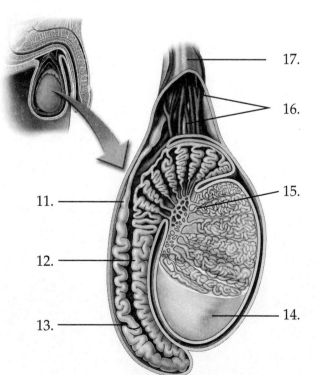

© Body Scientific International

(Continued)

Name _____ Date _____

Answer the following questions.

18. What is the main purpose of the male reproductive system?

_____

19. Which term describes the fertilization of the ovum?

_____

20. How are gametes different from other body cells?

_____

21. What are the two external components of the male reproductive system?

_____

22. Where do sperm mature until they are ready for fertilization?

_____

23. Why is it important that the testes are located outside of the abdominal cavity?

_____

24. Which hormone stimulates the testes to produce testosterone?

_____

25. What is the purpose of the flagellum?

_____

26. What is the main purpose of semen?

_____

27. What is the main purpose of the prostate gland?

_____

28. Which gland helps lubricate body surfaces during sexual intercourse?

_____

29. How does the penis become erect during sexual intercourse?

_____

30. Which internal anatomical structure of the male reproductive system is also considered part of the urinary system?

_____

Understanding Terms Related to Diseases and Conditions

Imagine that you are the radiologist at a children's hospital. You are reviewing the ultrasound results for a two-day old male patient. Determine the term for the patient's condition in each of the following situations.

1. the right testicle has not descended into the scrotal sac: _____

2. the left testicle is surrounded by a fluid-filled sac: _____

3. an abnormal enlargement of the vein in the spermatic cord of the right testicle: _____

Imagine that you are a nurse practitioner at a health clinic. Determine the diagnosis in the following cases.

4. a 23-year-old male comes into the clinic complaining of painful urination: _____

5. another male patient has discharge of pus from the end of his penis: _____

6. the shaft of another patient's penis has warts on it: _____

7. another patient is experiencing sores on the mucous membranes in his mouth, a rash on his hands and feet, sore throat, fatigue, and hair loss: _____

Imagine that you are a recent graduate who has been hired as a physician assistant at a rural health clinic that specializes in men's health. Your first patient of the day is Mr. Johnston, a 58-year-old male. Read the following descriptions and answer the accompanying questions.

8. Mr. Johnston has been complaining of having to urinate frequently. What is this condition called?

   _____

9. Mr. Johnston also tells you that it is difficult for him to start urinating. He feels like he "needs to go," but then it takes him longer to empty his bladder than it used to take. Which term describes the inability to completely empty the bladder?

   _____

10. You review Mr. Johnston's recent lab work and notice that his PSA is WNL. What does the PSA test measure?

    _____

11. You perform a DRE. What is this procedure?

    _____

12. You discover that Mr. Johnston's prostate gland is enlarged. What three medical terms can be used to describe this condition?

    _____

13. Why is Mr. Johnston having difficulty urinating?

    _____

(Continued)

Imagine that you are the medical assistant for Dr. Henrietta Haines, a reproductive endocrinologist who specializes in infertility. Read the following scenarios and answer the accompanying questions.

14. Dr. Haines sees many patients who are struggling with infertility. To meet the definition of infertility, for how long must a couple have practiced unprotected sex and been unable to achieve pregnancy?

   _____

15. When Dr. Haines interviews a couple, she will ask them about their own personal health histories, including the diagnosis and treatment of STIs and any other medical conditions. Which condition involves the abnormal location of the testis or testicles at birth that can affect a man's fertility after puberty?

   _____

16. Which medical term describes a problem with the spermatic cord that can affect a man's fertility?

   _____

17. Lab tests are routinely performed on a man's sperm to identify any potential causes of infertility. Which condition is characterized by a low sperm count?

   _____

Imagine that you are a registered nurse working in an oncology department as a patient education specialist. Your supervisor has asked you to develop a seminar for men. You know that it is important to present information that is relevant to the audience. Answer the following questions, which address important health issues for men.

18. There are specific types of cancer that affect men. What is the most common type of cancer in men older than 50 years of age?

   _____

19. You decide to also emphasize the importance of TSE. What type of cancer is determined during this procedure?

   _____

20. Accidents that occur during recreational sports may cause serious injury to the spermatic cord, which can cut off the blood supply to the testes. Which term describes this condition?

   _____

Analyzing Diagnostic- and Treatment-Related Terms

Match each of the following word parts with the correct meaning. You will not use all of the meanings.

_____ 1. trans-

_____ 2. vener/o

_____ 3. cauter/o

_____ 4. rect/o

_____ 5. -ion

_____ 6. -pexy

_____ 7. -al

_____ 8. circum-

_____ 9. -stomy

_____ 10. cis/o

A. pertaining to
B. rectum
C. around
D. to cut
E. across
F. surgical fixation
G. sexual contact
H. surgical opening
I. heat; burn
J. process; state; condition
K. beyond; excess

Answer the following questions.

11. A patient named Mr. Lee presents with c/o dysuria and polyuria. He has been diagnosed with BPH, and his PSA is WNL. What does this mean?

_____

_____

12. To help diagnose Mr. Lee's condition, the doctor orders a test that delivers sound waves to the pelvic area. What is the name of this test?

_____

13. The urologist recommends a TRUS for Mr. Lee. Describe this procedure.

_____

14. It is determined that Mr. Lee does not have prostate cancer. However, since Mr. Lee is experiencing dysuria and polyuria, the urologist recommends a procedure in which a section of the prostate gland is removed through the urethra. What is the name of this procedure?

_____

15. During preop instructions, the doctor tells Mr. Lee that he will have a Foley catheter placed into his bladder during the procedure, and that he will possibly go home with it for a few days. What is this device?

_____

_____

16. After the procedure, the recovery room nurse monitors Mr. Johnston for hematuria. Describe this condition.

_____

(Continued)

17. Which surgical procedure is often performed on newborn males to remove the foreskin of the penis?

   _____

18. The removal of the foreskin is recommended to reduce the risk of which three conditions?

   _____

   _____

19. Which surgical procedure is performed to secure an undescended testis into the scrotal sac?

   _____

20. What is the general term for a surgical procedure that can involve electrocautery or cryosurgery, and which is often performed to remove a cancerous area of the prostate gland?

   _____

21. Which two terms describe the procedure in which needles are inserted into the prostate gland to direct radio waves that aid in shrinking the prostate gland?

   _____

22. Which surgical procedure involves the removal of the entire prostate gland, as well as the seminal vesicles and surrounding tissue?

   _____

23. What is the purpose of TFT testing?

   _____

   _____

24. Which surgical procedure, when performed on a man, results in sterilization?

   _____

25. Which term describes the reversal of the procedure described in the previous question?

   _____

Preparing for Your Future in Healthcare

Imagine that you are the manager of a large hospital's human resources department. You have been asked to revise the organization's employee job descriptions. Using the information on page 380 of your textbook, list the job tasks and educational requirements for each of the following healthcare professionals.

1. Surgical Technician

   Typical Tasks:

   _____

   _____

   _____

   _____

   Educational Requirements:

   _____

   _____

2. Pharmacist

   Typical Tasks:

   _____

   _____

   _____

   _____

   Educational Requirements:

   _____

   _____

3. Oncologist

   Typical Tasks:

   _____

   _____

   _____

   _____

   Educational Requirements:

   _____

   _____

Chapter 13 Practice Test

Using the word parts on pages 363–364 of your textbook, identify the medical term that corresponds to each of the following definitions.

1. excision of the vas deferens (vessel; duct): _____

2. inflammation of the epididymis: _____

3. inflammation of the glans penis: _____

4. excessive flow from the prostate gland: _____

Break down each medical term listed below by rewriting the term, and then placing a slash between each word part (prefix, root word, combining vowel, and suffix if used). Then define each term.

5. phimosis

Breakdown: _____

Define: _____

6. gonorrhea

Breakdown: _____

Define: _____

7. varicocele

Breakdown: _____

Define: _____

8. hyperplasia

Breakdown: _____

Define: _____

9. orchiectomy

Breakdown: _____

Define: _____

10. transrectal

Breakdown: _____

Define: _____

(Continued)

Name _____ Date _____

Answer the following questions.

11. In which structure does spermatogenesis take place?

_____

12. What is another name for sperm?

_____

13. Which term describes a developing, fertilized ovum?

_____

14. Which term describes the period of time in which secondary sexual characteristics become evident?

_____

15. Are sperm cells larger or smaller than ovum cells?

_____

16. Where are sperm stored until they are transported through the vas deferens?

_____

Match each of the following diseases or conditions with the correct meaning. You will not use all of the meanings.

_____ 17. epididymitis

_____ 18. varicocele

_____ 19. oligospermia

_____ 20. trichomoniasis

_____ 21. prostatomegaly

_____ 22. anorchia

_____ 23. cryptorchidism

_____ 24. latent syphilis

_____ 25. azoospermia

_____ 26. prostatitis

_____ 27. herpes genitalis

_____ 28. testicular torsion

A. condition of one or two undescended testicles

B. abnormal enlargement of a vein in the spermatic cord

C. infection of the skin and mucosa of the genitals caused by HSV

D. benign prostatic hyperplasia (BPH)

E. absence of sperm in the semen

F. STI caused by the human papillomavirus

G. inflammation of the epididymis

H. condition of an abnormally low sperm count

I. stage of a chronic STI in which there may be no symptoms

J. sexually transmitted infection (STI) caused by a parasite

K. condition caused by the twisting of the spermatic cord

L. inflammation of the prostate

M. congenital absence of one or both testes

(Continued)

Identify the term that corresponds to each test described below.

29. involves palpation of the prostate to check for hypertrophy:

_____

30. performed by a male to self-check for abnormalities of the testes:

_____

31. measures the amount of sugar in the blood after a person has not eaten for at least 12 hours:

_____

32. used to screen pregnant females for syphilis:

_____

33. used to evaluate a male's fertility related to his semen:

_____

34. involves the evaluation of the tissue of the prostate gland:

_____

35. isolates and identifies bacteria that may be causing various infections:

_____

Identify the term that corresponds to each treatment described below.

36. drugs used to treat impotence:

_____

37. surgery to correct chronic phimosis:

_____

38. surgery to correct cryptorchidism:

_____

39. surgery to repair a varicocele:

_____

40. surgery to treat testicular cancer which involves removal of a testis:

_____

Chapter 14

The Female Reproductive System

Name _____ Date _____

Understanding Word Parts

Match each of the following word parts with the correct meaning. You will not use all of the meanings.

_____ 1. primi-

_____ 2. -arche

_____ 3. -gravida

_____ 4. nulli-

_____ 5. -partum

_____ 6. -rrhaphy

_____ 7. neo-

_____ 8. ante-

_____ 9. -para

_____ 10. -cyesis

A. new
B. to bear (offspring)
C. before
D. beginning
E. pregnant
F. abnormal condition
G. suture
H. no; none
I. state of pregnancy
J. first
K. childbirth

_____ 11. nat/i

_____ 12. ly/o

_____ 13. ligat/o

_____ 14. oophor/o

_____ 15. lact/o

_____ 16. dilat/o

_____ 17. colp/o

_____ 18. episi/o

_____ 19. salping/o

_____ 20. top/o

A. milk
B. ovary
C. fallopian tube
D. vagina
E. breakdown; dissolve; loosen
F. to bind
G. lump; mass
H. place; location; thing
I. vulva
J. to enlarge or expand
K. birth

(Continued)

Name _____ Date _____

Use the following combining forms and suffixes listed on pages 386–388 of your textbook to build the medical term that corresponds to each of the following definitions.

21. Word part: mast/o

    Definition: removal of a breast

    Term: _____

22. Word part: mamm/o

    Definition: process of recording a breast

    Term: _____

23. Word part: -ion

    Definition: process of binding or tying

    Term: _____

24. Word part: -cyesis

    Definition: state of a false pregnancy

    Term: _____

Break down each of the following medical terms by rewriting the term, and then placing a slash between each word part (prefix, root word, combining vowel, and suffix if used). Then define each term.

25. hysterosalpingogram

    Breakdown: _____

    Define: _____

26. vulvovaginitis

    Breakdown: _____

    Define: _____

27. gynopathy

    Breakdown: _____

    Define: _____

28. hysteropexy

    Breakdown: _____

    Define: _____

29. oligomenorrhea

    Breakdown: _____

    Define: _____

30. salpingo-oophorectomy

    Breakdown: _____

    Define: _____

Interpreting Medical Records

Read the following medical record and identify the meanings of the abbreviations and terms that appear in bold.

<u>Morning Glory Women's Health Clinic</u>

Patient Name: Rose Williams

Date of Birth: 7-4-1969

Medical Record No.: 35791

Date of Exam: 8-14-2017

Subjective Data: Pt is a 48 y/o female with extensive **gynecology** hx. **Menarche** occurred at age 13. Episode of **TSS** occurred at age 17, requiring hospitalization for three weeks. Pt received Dx of **cervical dysplasia** at age 18. Tx with **conization**. Subsequent **Pap tests** have been **WNL**. Pt married at age 20. Husband passed away six months ago at age 49 of prostate cancer. Pt has not been sexually active for the past 4 years. Pt is gravida 4, para 2, **AB** 2. Obstetrical hx includes spontaneous AB x 2 at ages 23 and 24. **D&C** was performed after each miscarriage. At age 25, Pt had a normal vaginal delivery of a live male by **CNM**. At age 27, Pt had **CS** of a live female by **OB/GYN** due to **breech birth**. Pt started on **OCPs** after the delivery of her second child but stopped taking them at age 30 due to excessive wt gain and **HA**. Pt's husband had **vasectomy** performed. Pt began experiencing severe pelvic pain at age 32. Exploratory **laparotomy** performed and diagnosis of **ovarian cyst** and **endometriosis** confirmed. Symptoms subsided about six months after procedure. Pt had experienced normal periods after laparotomy, but in the past six years she has developed increasingly irregular periods, **dysmenorrhea**, **oligomenorrhea**, and breakthrough bleeding between periods. Recent pelvic ultrasound revealed **PCOS** and **uterine fibroid** tumors. Pt's mother and sister have both had hysterectomies due to uterine cancer.

Objective Data: wt: 185 lb; ht: 64"; P: 80 bpm; **R**: 15; **T**: 98.6°; BP: 136/78

PE: **HEENT**: **PERRLA**, no mass or **adenomegaly**. **Palpation** of thyroid glands showed no lesions. Excessive hair growth noted on lower jaw line, extending down onto neck.

CV: Heart rate and rhythm normal, good capillary refill of digits

GU: Abdomen palpated, no obvious lesions or abnormalities noted. Well-healed lower lateral incision noted. Visual exam of perineum reveals well-healed **episiotomy** scar. Internal pelvic examination reveals enlarged ovaries, R>L. Uterus is tender during palpation, approximately six weeks size.

Assessment: PCOS with **hirsutism** and uterine fibroids

Plan: **TAH-BSO**; refer to endocrinology for **HRT postop**

---

1. gynecology: _____

   _____

2. menarche: _____

   _____

3. TSS: _____

4. cervical dysplasia: _____

   _____

5. conization: _____

   _____

6. Pap tests: _____

   _____

7. WNL: _____

8. AB: _____

9. D&C: _____

(Continued)

Name _____ Date _____

10. CNM: _____   22. PCOS: _____

11. CS: _____   23. uterine fibroids: _____

12. OB/GYN: _____   _____

13. breech birth: _____   24. R: _____

_____   25. T: _____

14. OCPs: _____   26. HEENT: _____

15. HA: _____   27. PERRLA: _____

16. vasectomy: _____   28. adenomegaly: _____

_____   _____

17. laparotomy: _____   29. palpation: _____

_____   _____

18. ovarian cyst: _____   30. episiotomy: _____

_____   _____

19. endometriosis: _____   31. hirsutism: _____

_____   _____

20. dysmenorrhea: _____   32. TAH-BSO: _____

_____   _____

21. oligomenorrhea: _____   33. HRT: _____

_____   34. postop: _____

Answer the following questions.

35. What was the probable cause of the patient's diagnosis and hospitalization at age 17?

_____

36. What was the probable cause of the patient's diagnosis of cervical dysplasia at age 18?

_____

37. How many times has Mrs. Williams been pregnant?

_____

38. What might cause the doctor to suspect that Mrs. Williams has hirsutism?

_____

39. Why does Mrs. Williams have a lower lateral incision on her abdomen?

_____

40. Why does Mrs. Williams have an episiotomy scar on her perineum?

_____

Comprehending Anatomy and Physiology Terminology

Identify the term that corresponds to each of the following descriptions.

1. the female sex cell: _____

2. the structure in which a female sex cell matures: _____

3. the gland in the brain that facilitates function of the ovaries: _____

4. the two hormones secreted by the ovaries: _____

5. the phase of development in which the sexual organs mature: _____

6. the structures located on the ends of the fallopian tubes that help direct the ova: _____

7. the muscular contraction and relaxation that helps move the ovum to the uterus: _____

8. the top of the uterus: _____

9. the outermost layer of the uterus: _____

10. the area where pubic hair is located: _____

11. the female erectile tissue: _____

12. the ducts that carry breast milk to the nipples: _____

13. the darker-colored circle around the nipple of the breast: _____

Answer the following questions.

14. When is the fertilized ovum considered an embryo?

_____

_____

15. When is the embryo considered a fetus?

_____

16. What does the term *gestation* mean?

_____

17. What does the term *effacement* mean?

_____

18. What is the purpose of the labia?

_____

19. How is colostrum different from regular breast milk?

_____

(Continued)

Name _____   Date _____

Label the different structures associated with a developing fetus in the following image.

20. _____
21. _____
22. _____
23. _____
24. _____
25. _____
26. _____
27. _____

20.
21.
22.
23.
24.
25.
26.
27.

© Body Scientific International

Answer the following questions.

28. What is the typical length of a human's gestation period?

_____

29. How is the first trimester defined?

_____

30. How is the second trimester defined? The third?

_____

_____

31. What three major events occur during the first stage of labor?

_____

32. In what position do most babies travel through the birth canal?

_____

33. What occurs during the third stage of labor?

_____

Name _____ Date _____

Understanding Terms Related to Diseases and Conditions

Imagine that you are a registered nurse for a large OB/GYN practice. You are reviewing the scheduled patients for the day so that you can prepare the rooms and necessary equipment for each appointment. Read each of the following scenarios and answer the accompanying questions.

1. The first patient is Linda Overton, a 54 y/o G3 P3 AB0. Mrs. Overton has c/o dysuria, frequent UTIs, and incontinence. On her previous visit, Mrs. Overton was diagnosed with a hernia of the bladder that bulges through the anterior vaginal wall, and a hernia of the rectum that bulges through the posterior vaginal wall. During this appointment, the doctor will prepare Mrs. Overton for surgery. What are the two preop dx for this patient?

   _____

2. The next patient is Amber Gray, a 25 y/o G0 P0 who has been experiencing pelvic pain and cramping, and who has been unable to get pregnant. The doctor suspects that Amber has endometrial tissue that has developed outside of her uterus. The doctor is going to schedule her for an exploratory laparoscopy. What is this patient's preop dx?

   _____

3. You notice that Rosa Longoria is scheduled to come in. You remember talking to her several months ago when she called the office with c/o mastodynia. Last week, she had her routine mammogram, and the radiologist reported several fibrous tumors in both breasts, which did not appear to be cancerous. The radiologist recommended evaluation for possible treatment options. What is the preliminary diagnosis for Mrs. Longoria?

   _____

4. The last patient of the day is Rachel Edmondson, a 54 y/o G6 P5 AB0. She made the appointment because she feels like her "insides are falling out into her vagina." She also complains of difficulty with urination, incontinence, and chronic yeast infection. Which term describes Mrs. Edmondson's yeast infection?

   _____

5. You suspect that Mrs. Edmondson's uterus is displaced due to weakened ligaments that normally hold it in place. Which term describes this condition?

   _____

Imagine that you are a nurse practitioner at a prenatal clinic. Read the following scenarios and answer the accompanying questions.

6. Trisha, a 16 y/o G2 P0 AB2 who is in for a follow-up on her recent Pap test, is in room one. She came to the clinic to get a prescription for birth control pills. Her Pap test came back positive for cervical dysplasia. When you explain this condition to Trisha, which virus will you say is the common cause?

   _____

7. How is this virus spread?

   _____

(Continued)

8. What is another uncomfortable condition that can be caused by this virus?

_____

9. If cervical dysplasia is not treated, which serious complication may occur?

_____

10. Nona, a 25 y/o G1 P1 AB0 who has been undergoing treatment for chlamydia, is in room two. Nona has been experiencing pelvic pain for several months now. What condition do you suspect Nona has?

_____

11. What is an additional complication of this condition that can affect the fallopian tubes and result in infertility?

_____

Imagine that you are the medical assistant at a women's clinic. Read the following scenarios and answer the accompanying questions.

12. The first patient you place in a room is Janice, a 25 y/o G5 P0 AB4 who is seeing the doctor for her six-week prenatal visit. Janice has a hx of spontaneous AB. Her first pregnancy ended at four weeks, her second ended at five weeks, and her third and fourth each ended at six weeks. Janice is very anxious about this visit. Her recent ultrasound showed the placenta was implanted at the lower end of the uterus. What is the medical term used to describe this condition?

_____

13. The next patient you place in a room is Chloe, a 35 y/o G1 P0 AB1. Chloe has been trying to get pregnant for 10 years and has experienced one spontaneous AB at five weeks gestation. Chloe wants to explore tx options for her infertility, but she is concerned because she had a friend whose zygote implanted in the fallopian tube, nearly resulting in death. What is the medical term for her friend's condition?

_____

14. The next patient is Felicia, an 18 y/o G2 P1 AB0 who is in the late second trimester of her second pregnancy. Felicia tells you that she has been having severe headaches, and that her feet and ankles are much more swollen than they were in her first pregnancy. Her BP is 160/98, which you know is much higher than normal. You collect a urine specimen from Felicia, and the UA shows protein in her urine. What is the possible diagnosis for Felicia's condition?

_____

15. Another patient, Veronica, brings her baby into the clinic for a four-month check up. The baby has been closely monitored by the neonatologist because he spent the first month of his life in the neonatal intensive care unit after aspirating early feces before delivery. Which term describes this condition?

_____

Analyzing Diagnostic- and Treatment-Related Terms

Read each of the following scenarios and answer the accompanying questions.

1. Mary is a 34 y/o G0 P0 who has been unable to get pregnant for over three years. The physician assistant orders a radiograph imaging procedure to determine whether there is any blockage of Mary's fallopian tubes. What is the name of this procedure?

   _____

2. The PA starts Mary on a medication that stimulates ovulation. What is the classification of this drug?

   _____

3. Six months after this test was performed, Mary makes an appointment to see the PA with c/o amenorrhea for two months. The PA performs a blood test that determines the presence of HCG. Mary's HCG test comes back positive. What is the name of this test, and what does a positive result mean?

   _____

   _____

4. Because Mary is almost 35 y/o, and she has a sister who had a baby with Down syndrome, the PA recommends that Mary have a test in which part of the placenta will be removed and evaluated for chromosomal defects. This test will be performed when Mary is 10–12 weeks pregnant. What is the name of this test?

   _____

5. This test comes back negative. However, because of the risk of genetic problems in children of older women, the PA recommends another test that will examine the amniotic fluid surrounding the baby. This test will be performed between 15 and 18 weeks gestation. What is the name of this test?

   _____

6. As Mary gets closer to her due date, the baby is turned so that the buttocks are closest to the birth canal. The PA instructs Mary about possibly delivering the baby by an incision through the abdominal wall and uterus. What is the name of this procedure?

   _____

7. One week before Mary's due date, the baby turns in the uterus so that the head is down and ready to go through the birth canal. When Mary is four days past her due date, the PA decides to schedule her and her husband to come into the labor and delivery ward of the hospital. At this time, the PA starts Mary on a medication that will stimulate labor and start her contractions. What is the name of this medication?

   _____

(Continued)

8. During this stage of labor, Mary is fitted with an electronic device that records the baby's heart rate and rhythm. What is the name of this procedure?

_____

9. Mary's labor starts and her cervix is 100% effaced and dilated. As the baby begins to crown, the obstetrician in the L&D makes an incision into the perineum to prevent tearing. What is the name of this procedure?

_____

10. Mary's PA visits her in the postpartum care area of the birthing unit at the hospital. Mary is bonding well with the baby, her colostrum has come in, and the baby is nursing well. Mary and her husband do not want another baby, so they all discuss birth control measures. The PA offers to give Mary a prescription for a medication that will prevent ovulation. What is the classification of this medication?

_____

11. Frances is a 45 y/o G3 P2 AB1 who comes to the gynecologist's office for a follow-up appointment. The nurse practitioner interviews Frances about her health issues. Frances tell her that she is recently divorced and has become sexually active with several partners in the past nine months. The NP asks Frances if she examines her breasts at least once a month to check for any changes. What is this examination called?

_____

12. The NP recommends that Frances have a radiographic examination of her breasts to check for any cancer or other changes. What is the name of this test?

_____

13. Next, the NP prepares Frances for a manual and visual examination of the external and internal female organs. What is the name of this test?

_____

14. Frances tells the NP that she has been having pelvic pain in the area of her right ovary. The NP palpates this area and is concerned about an abnormality. The NP orders a test that uses ultrasonic sound waves to produce an image of a structure in the pelvic cavity. What is the name of this test?

_____

15. Two weeks after these tests, Frances returns to the clinic for a follow-up. The test of her cervical cells came back positive for cervical dysplasia. The NP recommends that Frances tell her sexual partners about this diagnosis. Why is it important for her to notify them of her condition?

_____

_____

_____

(Continued)

16. The NP performs a visual examination of the vagina and cervix with a scope and takes more samples of the tissue of the cervix. What is the name of this procedure?

_____

17. This test comes back positive for cervical cancer. The NP refers Frances to a gynecological oncologist for further evaluation and treatment. The GYN specialist examines Frances' cervix and determines that she needs several procedures. There is one area of diseased tissue on the cervix that she determines can be removed by excising a cone-shaped section. What is the name of this procedure?

_____

18. The GYN specialist decides to remove a small portion of another area on the cervix so that it can be examined under a microscope for further evaluation. What is the name of this procedure?

_____

19. The results of the ultrasound test used to evaluate the right ovary also showed a questionable area on the uterus. The GYN specialist determines that a sample of the endometrial tissue of Frances' uterus needs to be excised so it can be tested for uterine cancer. What is the name of this procedure?

_____

20. These tests come back positive for cervical and uterine cancer. The GYN specialist informs Frances that she will need to have a surgical procedure in which the cervix, uterus, both ovaries, and both fallopian tubes are removed through an incision in the abdomen. What is the name of this procedure?

_____